Arthritis

Your comprehensive guide to pain management, medication, diet, exercise, surgery, and physical therapies

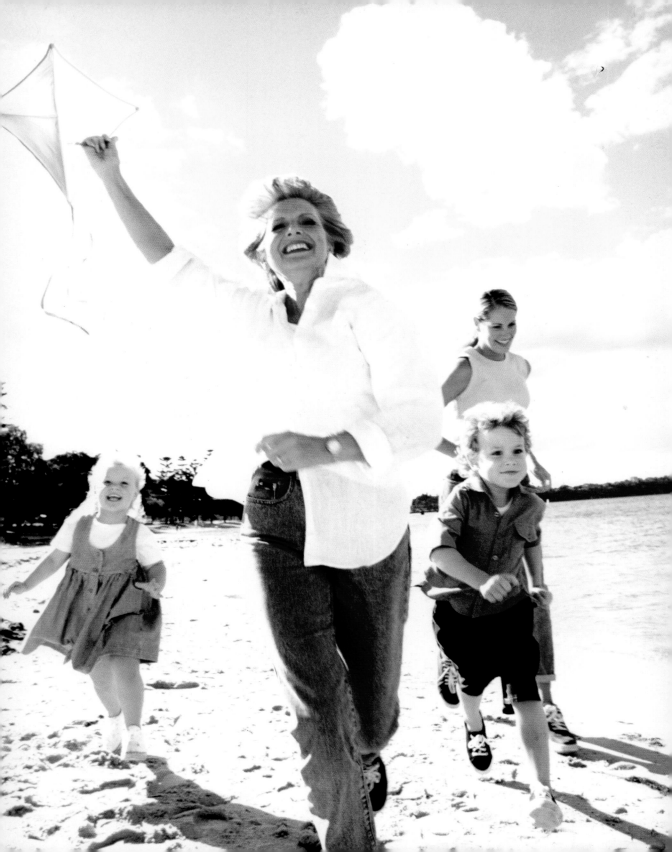

Arthritis

Your comprehensive guide to pain management, medication, diet, exercise, surgery, and physical therapies

Howard Bird, Caroline Green, Andrew Hamer,
Alison Hammond, Janet Harkess, Mike Hurley,
Paula Jeffreson, Dorothy Pattison, David L. Scott
US Consultant: Robin K. Dore, MD

London, New York, Munich, Melbourne, Delhi

Senior Editor Janet Mohun
US Senior Editor Jill Hamilton
Editor Pip Morgan
Designer Phil Gamble
Senior Art Editor Helen Spencer
Executive Managing Editor Adèle Hayward
Managing Art Editor Karla Jennings
DTP Designer Traci Salter
Picture Researcher Andrea Sadler
Medical Illustrator Philip Wilson
Production Controller Luca Frassinetti

This edition first published in the United States in 2006 by
DK Publishing, Inc., 375 Hudson Street, New York, New York 10014

06 07 08 09 10 9 8 7 6 5 4 3 2 1

A CIP catalog record for this book is available from the Library of Congress.
ISBN 0-7566-1870-3
Reproduced by Colourscan, Singapore
Printed and bound in Singapore by Star Standard

Discover more at
www.dk.com

Foreword

Arthritis is a term that actually describes more than 100 different diseases. As a rheumatologist treating patients with arthritis, I see people affected in many different ways. No two cases of rheumatoid arthritis are exactly alike. No two people with osteoarthritis have the same experience. Regardless, physicians like me treat all patients the same—with individual focus and concern, and with a goal to educate them about their arthritis so together we can improve the quality of their lives.

In the not so distant past, a patient receiving an arthritis diagnosis might have replied, "Well, I guess there is nothing I can do about it." Thankfully, that is no longer the case. Innovative treatment options, including biologic drugs and improved surgical techniques, have dramatically improved the outlook for people with arthritis. Other "innovations" have been renewed emphasis on appropriate physical activity, patient self-management (like stress management, weight loss, and joint protection), and patient-physician communication. Today, we want the patient to be a partner in arthritis management. We want patients today and in the future to say, "I can do something about my arthritis."

To be a partner in his or her arthritis care, a person with arthritis needs to know about the disease, the management options, and much more. Resources like this book, in addition to the information, programs, and support provided by the Arthritis Foundation throughout the United States, help people with arthritis realize that they are far from alone, educate them about their chronic disease, and help them, working in partnership with their physicians, to manage and take control of their arthritis.

I hope you will use these resources, become well-informed about your condition, and feel you can do something about your arthritis.

Robin K. Dore MD

ROBIN K. DORE MD
CLINICAL PROFESSOR OF MEDICINE,
DAVID GEFFEN SCHOOL OF MEDICINE AT UCLA,
LOS ANGELES, CA
PRIVATE PRACTICE, ANAHEIM, CA

Contents

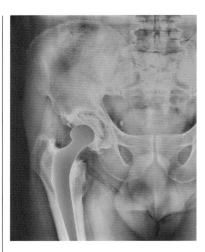

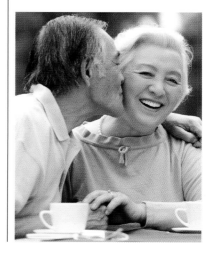

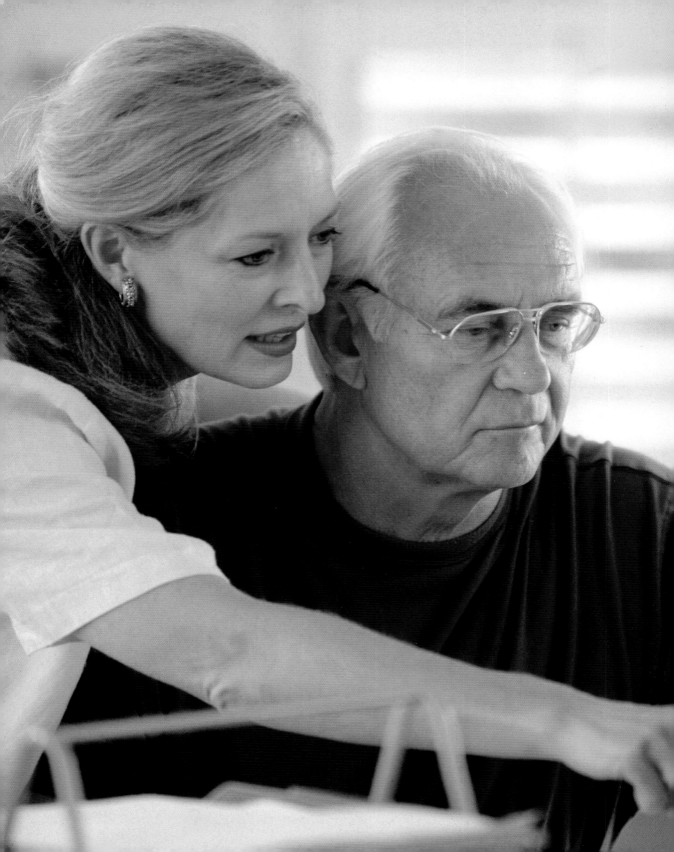

What is arthritis?

In the last 50 years our understanding of
arthritis has improved enormously. Where
once it was seen as one condition, it is now
known to be a group of almost 200. This
knowledge has helped doctors to be more
specific about diagnosing the type of arthritis
and to be able to devise treatments for
individual people.

We still don't know what causes arthritis,
although we have a much better idea of the
risk factors involved—from inheritance and
gender to obesity and infections. As a result,
we are better able to know who is likely to
develop one or other of the arthritic conditions.

Improvements in diagnosis have
accompanied innovations in scanning
techniques, so arthritis can now be detected
earlier and with more precision. Specialized
healthcare professionals and organizations
capable of helping you with your arthritis have
grown in number and expertise. They all agree
that people with arthritis who communicate
well with their physicians and specialists stand
a better chance of successfully managing
their condition.

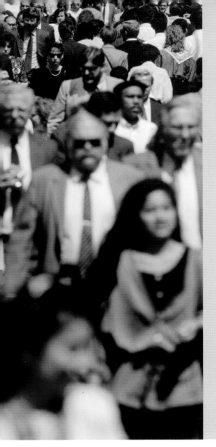

Understanding Arthritis

Arthritis is not a single disease but a number of different disorders that can affect the joints at any stage of life, from the early days of childhood until the closing stages of old age. Arthritis has two key characteristics—joint pain and inflammation. Some people with arthritis only have pain but most have a combination of the two. To make sense of arthritis it is important to understand some key general information, such as the types of joints and the causes and consequences of joint inflammation.

Anyone can develop arthritis. It affects men and women of all ages, and sometimes even children.

The characteristics of arthritis

The hallmark of arthritis is joint inflammation, which leads to tenderness and swelling. People with arthritis usually complain of joint stiffness as well.

The many types of arthritis can be divided into inflammatory and degenerative groups, although the distinction is not always clear-cut. In inflammatory arthritis, such as rheumatoid arthritis, there is more swelling of the soft tissues around a joint, and stiffness is most noticeable in the morning, when it may last an hour or more.

Degenerative arthritis, such as osteoarthritis, is characterized by more bony swelling and less soft-tissue swelling; stiffness usually occurs at rest or after exercise.

When only one joint is involved the condition is sometimes called a monoarthritis. When many joints are affected the condition may be described as a polyarthritis. Oligoarthritis is sometimes used to describe a condition involving a few joints. One feature of some forms of arthritis is that similar joints are involved on both sides of the body. This symmetrical joint involvement is very typical of rheumatoid arthritis.

Are women usually more affected by arthritis than men?

Yes. It is mainly due to the fact that impaired immunity is a significant factor. Most medical conditions in which there is impaired immunity are three times more common in women. However, other diseases, such as ankylosing spondylitis and gout, are more common in men.

Which joints are affected?

Most forms of arthritis affect the small joints in the hands and feet and the large joints of the knees and hips, although any joint can be involved.

Different forms of arthritis affect different joints. Osteoarthritis, for example, usually affects the top two joints of the fingers and the base of the thumb, as well as the knees and the hips. Rheumatoid arthritis usually involves the bottom two joints of the fingers and thumbs, and also the wrists. Gout characteristically affects the joint at the base of the big toe.

Challenges to overcome

People with arthritis often have to face difficulties and challenges that can compromise their way of life, although many of these can also be overcome.

There are four main reasons for these challenges. First, the pain and inflammation immediately limit what you can do. Second, the progressive damage to your joints makes your muscles weak, making you less active. Third, the chronic pain wears you out and restricts the amount of exercise you are able to do. Finally, the conditions that are commonly associated with arthritis can put a strain on your quality of life.

Many forms of arthritis, especially rheumatoid arthritis, are associated with changes in the skin or internal organs because they affect all the systems in the body, not just locally in the joints.

Who is affected by arthritis?

Anyone can develop arthritis. It affects men and women of all ages, and sometimes even children (see p.182). No one knows for sure

A COMMON CONDITION
Arthritis is a common condition in countries throughout the world and most characteristically affects people in later life.

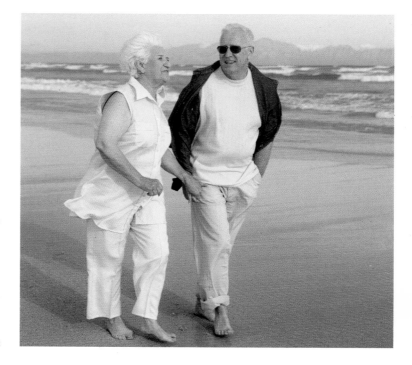

TYPES OF JOINTS

Joints are the sites in the body where two bones make contact. Most joints have a space called the synovial cavity between the two bones. These synovial joints, such as the hip and elbow, allow movement and provide mechanical support.

Some joints, such as the joints of the spine, are connected by disks of cartilage and permit some movement; others, such as the bones of the skull, are bound by fibrous tissue and permit no movement at all. In general, the joints that allow movement are the joints involved in arthritis.

Although they are different, synovial joints share one underlying similarity: the surfaces of the two bones, where they meet, are covered in a thin superficial layer of tissue called the synovial membrane. Deeper layers of cartilage are able to absorb shocks.

Synovial joints move in various ways. Some, such as the wrist, have a wide range of movement but do not move far in any direction. Hinge joints, such as the elbow, allow plenty of movement but only in a single plane. Ball-and-socket joints, such as the hip, have a wide range of movement in several directions.

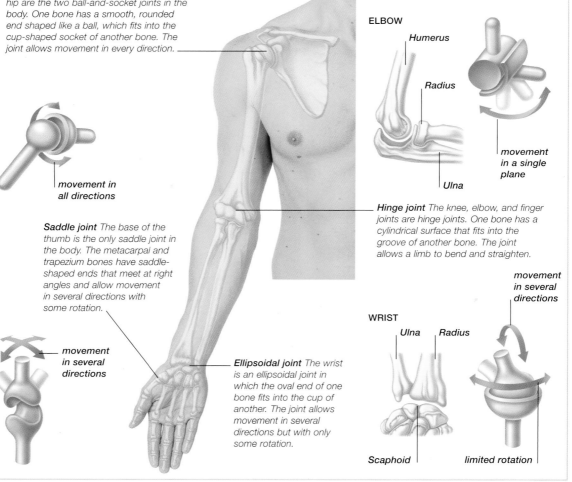

Ball-and-socket joint *The shoulder and hip are the two ball-and-socket joints in the body. One bone has a smooth, rounded end shaped like a ball, which fits into the cup-shaped socket of another bone. The joint allows movement in every direction.*

movement in
all directions

Saddle joint *The base of the thumb is the only saddle joint in the body. The metacarpal and trapezium bones have saddle-shaped ends that meet at right angles and allow movement in several directions with some rotation.*

movement
in several
directions

Ellipsoidal joint *The wrist is an ellipsoidal joint in which the oval end of one bone fits into the cup of another. The joint allows movement in several directions but with only some rotation.*

ELBOW

Humerus

Radius

Ulna

movement
in a single
plane

Hinge joint *The knee, elbow, and finger joints are hinge joints. One bone has a cylindrical surface that fits into the groove of another bone. The joint allows a limb to bend and straighten.*

movement
in several
directions

WRIST

Ulna   Radius

Scaphoid

limited rotation

why some people develop arthritis and others do not, but there is a great deal of information about who is most at risk. Depending on a range of genetic and environmental factors, you might be more likely than others to develop a particular type of arthritis. These risk factors vary between diseases and also differ between ages, sexes, and ethnic groups. (See individual types of arthritis in Chapter Two for more specific information.)

Arthritis usually affects people in later life, although this general rule is not as straightforward as it sounds for two reasons. First, arthritis, especially osteoarthritis, begins mainly in old age. Second, the arthritis that people develop at a younger age has a cumulative and longstanding effect over time.

What is inflammation?

The process of inflammation is the first response that our immune systems take to combat infection or to remove irritation. The response is essential to our survival because it helps us protect ourselves and deal with a wide range of unwanted risks, such as disease-causing bacteria. In the usual course of events, the inflammation dies down and the affected tissues return to normal.

Classically, inflammation has a quintet of features—redness, heat, swelling, pain, and loss of function. In arthritis, only swelling and pain are present to any great extent, with loss of function being an inevitable consequence.

Redness and heat are caused by an increased blood supply to a particular part of the body, such as a joint. Blood vessels upstream of the joint become wider, while those downstream are narrowed. These changes cause the inflamed joint to swell. White blood cells accumulate and release a variety of active materials into the inflamed joint. The combination of the tissue swelling and the active substances from the white cells make the joint painful.

THE HEALTHY JOINT

The cartilage and synovial fluid play an important role in the health of a joint. The cartilage protecting the ends of the bones has to be smooth, springy, and tough. The fluid provides the nutrients the cartilage needs to renew itself and filters out the debris as the surface layers of cartilage are worn away. The movement of the joint constantly presses and releases the cartilage like a sponge, allowing nourishment to reach the deeper layers of cartilage and waste to be removed.

SYNOVIAL JOINT
This cutaway shows the principal features of every synovial (freely movable) joint.

Bone

Cartilage

Synovial fluid lubricates the ends of the bones.

Cartilage covers the bone ends and prevents damage.

Synovial membrane secretes lubricating synovial fluid.

Fibrous capsule forms a protective casing for the joint

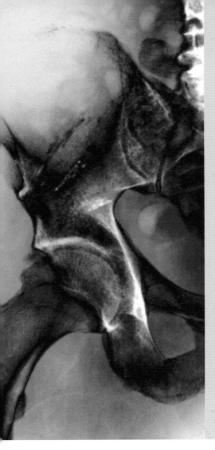

The main types of arthritis

Arthritis is very common, with more than 100 identifiable types. Only a few, however, such as osteoarthritis and rheumatoid arthritis, affect people in significant numbers. Arthritis develops in various settings and for a number of reasons: wear and tear of the bones in a joint; longstanding (chronic) inflammation of the soft tissues around a joint; genetic presdisposition; the accumulation of crystals in a joint; and an infection in a joint. As a result, many conditions are all categorized under the term arthritis.

Trauma or a major injury or operation on a joint may lead to osteoarthritis at that site later in life.

Osteoarthritis

Osteoarthritis is the most common form of arthritis. It is usually considered to be a degenerative "wear-and-tear" condition that is associated with aging, although younger people can also develop it following an injury.

If you have osteoarthritis you will probably find that only one joint or a small number of joints are affected. The most likely are the top joints of your fingers, the base joint of your thumb, your hips, or your knees.

Osteoarthritis is more common in the knee than in the hip; taken together, the hips and knees are affected in 10–20 percent of people aged over 65 and are a major cause of pain and disability in elderly people.

About 21 million people in the US have osteoarthritis, but only half of those actively seek treatment. The others do not know they have it, or suffer any pain, although it may be seen when they are X–rayed for other reasons.

Risk factors

Usually, several risk factors need to be present before osteoarthritis develops. The main factors include age, gender, obesity, occupation,

Q&A

Can changes in the weather make my osteoarthritis worse?

Cold wet weather may make your joints feel worse but there is no strong evidence to suggest that your osteoarthritis is affected. People often think that if they moved to a warm dry climate their arthritis would improve. However, osteoarthritis is just as common in warmer regions as in colder climates.

genetics, trauma, or any previous inflammation of a joint.

■ **AGE** is the dominant risk factor. Osteoarthritis usually starts after the late 40s and rises steeply with increasing age. Most people aged over 65 years have some evidence of osteoarthritis. As more people live longer, osteoarthritis will become more common, probably because they will experience increasing muscle weakness and they will be less able to repair worn or damaged tissues.

■ **GENDER** is important, too. For most joints, particularly the knees and hands, osteoarthritis is more common and more severe in women than in men.

■ **OBESITY** (more than 25 percent above a person's target healthy weight) markedly increases the risk of osteoarthritis. This is most likely because of pressure of the increased weight on the joints. The knee is at particular risk. At the same time, people who are

SITES OF ARTHRITIS

Osteoarthritis (opposite) and rheumatoid arthritis (see p.18) tend to affect certain joints, although any joint might be involved. The main joints affected by osteoarthritis are the hips, knees, hands, and feet. Rheumatoid arthritis targets a wider range of joints and varies considerably from one person to another. The hands and feet are often involved, as are the wrists, ankles, shoulders, and knees. Less commonly affected are the elbows, jaws, and bones in the neck.

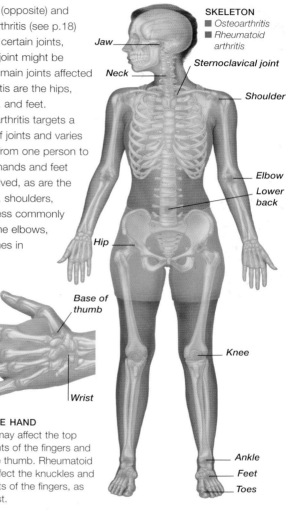

SKELETON
■ *Osteoarthritis*
■ *Rheumatoid arthritis*

Jaw
Neck
Sternoclavical joint
Shoulder
Elbow
Lower back
Hip
Base of thumb
Knee
Wrist
Ankle
Feet
Toes

JOINTS OF THE HAND
Osteoarthritis may affect the top and middle joints of the fingers and the base of the thumb. Rheumatoid arthritis may affect the knuckles and the middle joints of the fingers, as well as the wrist.

overweight or obese increase their chances of osteoarthritis worsening once it has developed.

■ **TRAUMA** or a major injury or operation on a joint may lead to osteoarthritis at that site later in life. If you do a hard and repetitive activity you may injure a joint and

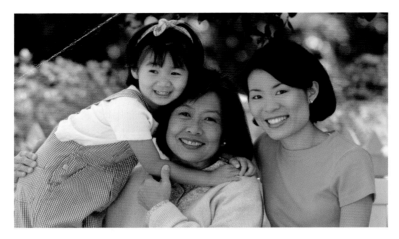

RUNNING IN THE FAMILY
Nodal osteoarthritis is a condition that may be inherited, particularly on the female side of the family.

In osteoarthritis, the surface of the cartilage breaks down and wears away so that the bones under the cartilage start to rub together.

make it prone to osteoarthritis. This condition may also develop in an injured joint if you exercise before the injury has had time to heal properly.

Occupations such as farming make osteoarthritis of the hip more likely; soccer players are prone to osteoarthritis of the knee. Occupations involving knee bending, squatting, and heavy lifting are associated with osteoarthritis of the knee.

■ **GENETICS** plays a clear role in the development of the common form of nodal osteoarthritis (see p.18), which particularly affects the hands of middle-aged women. In osteoarthritis of the knee and hip, heredity plays a smaller, although still significant, role. General osteoarthritis probably has a genetic basis too.

Genes that are likely to be involved in the common forms of osteoarthritis include the vitamin D receptor gene, the insulin-like growth factor genes, the cartilage

oligomeric protein genes, and the HLA region (see p.200). There are some very rare but dramatic forms of osteoarthritis that start at a young age and run in families. These are linked with single genes that affect the protein collagen, which is an essential component of healthy cartilage.

What happens?

Osteoarthritis often develops slowly and varies from person to person: some people have only minor symptoms, but in others the condition can be very severe.

The primary site is the cartilage that covers the ends of the bones in a joint. Healthy cartilage lets bones glide over one another and absorbs the energy from movement. In osteoarthritis, the surface of the cartilage breaks down and wears away so that the bones under the cartilage start to rub together. The results are pain, swelling, and reduced movement.

Q&A

Last winter, I fell and injured my knee while I was skiing—does this mean I may develop osteoarthrosis later in life?

Yes, it's possible, particularly if you damaged the cartilage. In addition, if you didn't wait for the injury to heal completely before you returned to physical exercise, you may have made it more likely that the joint will be affected by osteoarthritis—but no one can say when.

The swelling is usually the result of lumps forming on the bone but sometimes it can be caused by increased fluid in the joint. In some cases, the joint makes an abnormal noise, or crepitus, when it moves. Affected joints often stiffen after exercise, sometimes known as "gelling." Some people with osteoarthritis feel stiff in the morning, but this lasts only a few minutes. Osteoarthritis does not affect internal organs.

Eventually, the affected joint loses its normal shape and becomes deformed. Small spurs called osteophytes often form at the end of the bones. Small pieces of cartilage or bone may break off and float inside the joint space, causing further pain and damage. In some ways osteoarthritis represents joint failure, which can be minimal or complete, depending on its severity.

Osteoarthritis of the knee

When osteoarthritis affects the knee, particularly among people between their late 50s and early 70s, it can be very complicated. Osteoarthritis of the knee is more common in women than men and generally affects both knees.

You may have more chance of developing osteoarthritis of the knee if you are overweight, have osteoarthritis in another joint, or have had a previous sports injury or knee surgery, in particular cartilage removal.

Often, however, there is no obvious cause. Pain is usually felt at the front and sides of the knee. In the later stages, the knees can become bent and deformed.

Osteoarthritis of the hip

Women and men are equally affected by osteoarthritis of the hip. It can start in their 40s but

OSTEOARTHRITIS OF THE HIP

Mechanical wear and tear can cause the cartilage of the hip joint to deteriorate and unprotected bone to be exposed. As a result, the space between the head of the thigh bone and the socket of the pelvis narrows to the point where the two bones touch. Prolonged contact and damage leads to the development of bony spurs, or osteophytes. The hip becomes painful and restricted in its movements. Analgesics may bring some relief but serious cases will require surgery to replace the hip (see p.92).

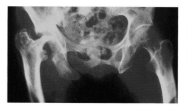

OSTEOARTHRITIC HIP
This X–ray of an osteoarthritic hip joint shows how the space between the head of the thigh bone and the socket in the pelvis has narrowed so much they are almost touching.

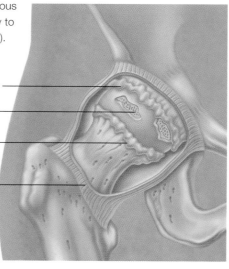

Osteophytes form on the socket of the pelvis.

Cartilage A hole leaves bone unprotected.

Osteophytes form on the head of the thigh bone.

Joint capsule Inflammation of the joint capsule may cause pain.

JOINT CAPSULE OF AN OSTEOARTHRITIC HIP

more usually later in life. One or both hips are equally likely to be involved. Certain hip problems that were present at birth or have developed in childhood may later lead to osteoarthritis. Some people have anatomical features that predispose them to osteoarthritis. For example, in certain cases, the acetabulum—the cup of the pelvic socket into which the head of the thigh bone sits—is not as well developed as it should be.

Hip pain from osteoarthritis is usually at the front of the groin, but it can also occur in the buttock or in the knee, when it is considered to be "referred" pain.

Osteoarthritis of the hands

This condition mainly involves women and commonly starts in the late 40s or early 50s, often around the time of menopause (see p.192). It chiefly affects the joint at the base of the thumbs and the joints at the top of the fingers. Although the fingers become knobbly and sometimes slightly bent, they work well and rarely cause long-term problems.

Nodal osteoarthritis affects the finger joints. These joints are swollen and tender, especially at the beginning, and then develop firm, bony, knobby swellings. When these affect the top joints of the fingers they are called Heberden's nodes, after the 18th century British physician who first described them.

In some cases, similar bony swellings—called Bouchard's nodes after the 19th century French pathologist—appear on the joints in the middle of the fingers. Occasionally, by the time these two types of node have formed, the joints are relatively free from pain and tenderness.

People with nodal osteoarthritis in middle age are more likely to develop osteoarthritis of the knee during old age.

Rheumatoid arthritis

About 2.1 million adults in the US have rheumatoid arthritis, making it the most common form of inflammatory arthritis. Although its cause is unknown, it is usually thought to be an autoimmune disease in which the body starts to attack itself—but the evidence for this is incomplete.

Rheumatoid arthritis can occur at any age, but it is more common in later life. Usually, many joints are involved (see p.15). It is a long-term (chronic) disease that is characterized by persistent joint inflammation. This, over a prolonged period of time, results in irreversible joint damage.

Risk factors

Gender, genetics, and age are the most important risk factors. Others include heavy smoking, obesity, a history of blood transfusions, and, in women, a shorter fertile period associated with low levels of reproductive hormones. Drinking coffee and trauma may also be predisposing risk factors, although the evidence is inconclusive.

■ **GENDER** is a dominant risk factor —up to three-quarters of people with rheumatoid arthritis are women. Research suggests that in a population of 100,000 adults there will be about 36 new cases of rheumatoid arthritis in women and 14 in men per year. The incidence of rheumatoid arthritis rises steeply as people grow older, especially in men.

■ **GENETICS** play a significant role in rheumatoid disease. Up to 60 percent of the predisposition to rheumatoid arthritis is explained by genetic factors (see p.200). The disease is strongly related to the presence of a protein on the surface of white blood cells (leucocytes) called HLA–DR4. Most evidence suggests that genetics contribute mainly to the severity of the disease rather than to disease susceptibility.

■ **AGE** has a complex effect on the risks of developing the disease, which can begin at any age. It was viewed traditionally as starting in young adulthood, with a peak age

RHEUMATOID ARTHRITIS OF THE HANDS

Rheumatoid arthritis usually affects a number of joints, often the same joints similarly—but not always simultaneously—on both sides of the body. Although the joints affected vary from person to person, several specific joints are more commonly involved than others. In the hand, these include the base of the thumb, the middle joints of the fingers, the knuckles, and the wrists.

As rheumatoid arthritis develops, the cartilage is damaged, and the joints swell and become inflamed, causing pain and restricted movement. Moving the hand may cause a creaking sound called crepitus. Eventually, the fingers bend away from the thumb.

Inflamed synovial membrane causes pain, swelling, and stiffness in the joint.

Damaged bone

Damaged cartilage exposes the bone and bony erosions appear.

Cartilage A hole in the cartilage exposes the bone.

Joint capsule swells and is painful

BASE OF THE THUMB

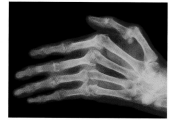

RHEUMATOID HAND
This X–ray of a left hand affected by severe rheumatoid arthritis shows the swollen and inflamed joints (orange) that are a feature of the disease. As the cartilage deteriorates, the bones of the joint become damaged.

of onset between 20 and 45 years. For unknown reasons, this has changed and the average age of onset has increased to 60 years.

What happens?

The synovial membrane of one or more joints becomes inflamed, causing pain, swelling, and stiffness. In the early stages, the swelling involves only soft tissue and there may be an an increase of fluid in the joint (an effusion).

Stiffness is characteristic of any type of inflammatory arthritis and is usually present in the morning—it can last for an hour or two, but in severe cases can persist all day. The inflammation spreads to the synovial sheaths that protect and lubricate the tendons linking the bones of the joints to the muscles that move them.

As the disease progresses, the inflammation persists for some unknown reason and results in progressive and usually irreversible damage to joints. The more the inflammation, the greater the risks of damage. Bony swellings appear and deformity develops as the joints become damaged and begin to fail. The muscles weaken, partly though lack of use and partly from the effects of a generalized inflammatory condition.

Rheumatoid arthritis starts in different ways. Usually, it starts slowly, with intermittent pain and swelling in some joints, especially in the fingers, wrists, and feet. The

symptoms gradually worsen until it is self-evident to the individual that there is something wrong with the joints. In perhaps 20 percent of cases, the disease starts very suddenly: one day the individual is normal and the next, many joints are painful, swollen, and stiff.

In some people the disease starts in less usual ways. For example, it may involve a single joint. In others, the disease comes and goes repeatedly, often over several years, before becoming persistent. Occasionally, it starts with pain and stiffness around the shoulders and mimics a condition called polymyalgia rheumatica.

The way the disease progresses is variable. Some people have a mild disease with few problems and can live normal lives. For others, the disease may enter a period of sustained remission without returning, or else follows an intermittent course, when flare-ups are followed by remissions that do not last long.

Many people have chronic persistent arthritis, in which continuing disease activity has added flare-ups from time to time. A few people have a persisting severe disease that remains active despite the best efforts of most therapies.

Disability

Taken together, inflammation and damage to joints cause marked disability. This varies with time and is unique to an individual, depending on the exact ways their joints are involved. Some people with rheumatoid arthritis are simply unable to do normal things. The disability is also psychological and social. For example, many, though by no means all, people with rheumatoid arthritis find it difficult to work and some will need to leave their job as a result. (See Day-to-Day Living, p.134.)

Ankylosing spondylitis

This inflammatory disease affects the spine predominantly and can result in marked stiffness or even fusion of the spine (see right). "Ankylosing" is another word for stiffening, while "spondylitis" means inflammation of the spine.

The cause of anklyosing spondylitis is unknown. Unlike rheumatoid arthritis the disorder is not associated with the presence of rheumatoid factor in the blood (see p.41); nor does it show any features of autoimmunity. The two sacroiliac joints, which connect the spine to the the pelvis and do not possess a synovium, are also involved.

At least 500,000 US adults have the disorder; most likely there are more because it is difficult to diagnose in its early stages, and is the most overlooked cause of back pain in young adults.

Risk factors

Genetics and gender are the main risk factors. It is sometimes related to infection so some experts think there may be an infectious trigger.

■ **GENETICS** A gene called HLA-B27 plays a role in the condition. Up to 95 percent of people with the condition have the gene, compared to less than 10 percent of the general population.

STIFFENING OF THE SPINE

In ankylosing spondyltis, the joints between the vertebrae of the spine become inflamed, starting at the sacroiliac joints where the spine links with the pelvis. The ligaments around the joints accumulate calcium salts and harden. New bone forms once the inflammation subsides. As a result, the spine stiffens and becomes inflexible. Eventually, in severe cases, the joints may fuse and prevent movement. The joints connecting the vertebrae to the ribs may become inflamed, which often makes breathing difficult.

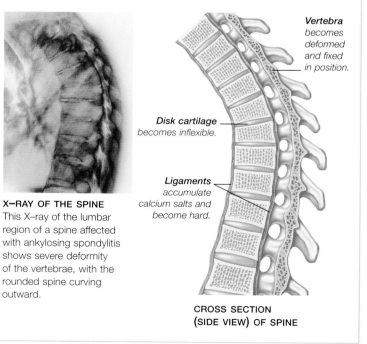

X–RAY OF THE SPINE
This X–ray of the lumbar region of a spine affected with ankylosing spondylitis shows severe deformity of the vertebrae, with the rounded spine curving outward.

Vertebra becomes deformed and fixed in position.

Disk cartilage becomes inflexible.

Ligaments accumulate calcium salts and become hard.

CROSS SECTION (SIDE VIEW) OF SPINE

■ **GENDER** is important; men are most often affected by the disease, particularly those in their 20s and 30s. The ratio of men to women with ankylosing spondylitis is about 5 to 1. When the disease affects women it tends to be milder than in men.

What happens?

The initial features of ankylosing spondylitis are stiffness, an ache in the lower back, and reduced movement of the spine. The stiffness is present in the morning and often lasts for several hours.

Some people with ankylosing spondylitis have only mild aches and pains that progress slowly over months or years. Others have a more active disease that leads to feelings of ill-health and fatigue, and to potential loss of weight.

In addition, the disorder is associated with iritis, which causes an acutely inflamed red eye and requires immediate medical attention to avoid permanent damage to the eye.

Over time, the disease may clear up or cause only minor stiffness; or it may become more serious as the stiffness progresses, with limited movement of the spine that results in a hunched posture, rounded spine, and a flat chest. Arthritis of other joints, such as the knee or hip, usually clears up with time. Only a very few patients develop a progressive destructive arthritis of their joints.

Psoriatic arthritis

Psoriatic arthritis is not a common disorder—around 160,000 adults in the US are affected. It is an inflammatory arthritis associated with the skin condition psoriasis, although this is not inevitable and, in most instances, is not usually a consequence. In fact, sometimes the arthritis develops first. About 1 in 50 people have psoriasis; of these, about 1 in 14 develop psoriatic arthritis.

Psoriatic arthritis affects men and women in equal measure and usually starts in middle age. The cause is unknown, although genetics probably play a part. Like ankylosing spondylitis, it may be triggered by an infection.

What happens?

Many people with psoriatic arthritis experience inflammation in one or two joints, such as a knee or ankle. In other people, it involves the top joint of the fingers (see left). Sometimes, many joints are affected and the disease is similar to rheumatoid arthritis.

About one third of people with psoriatic arthritis also have spinal disease, with back or neck pain due to spinal inflammation. Tendons and the site where tendons are attached to bones may also become inflamed. This can cause pain in the Achilles tendon, in the heels, and around the top of the thigh bone.

Gout

Gout is a disorder with a clearly identified cause—the presence of uric acid crystals in the synovial fluid of a joint. Gout affects the joints, particularly in the big toe, where it can be very painful. In fact, in an acute attack, gout can be the most painful arthritis of all.

Gout is a disorder of the metabolism of uric acid. It affects approximately 2.1 million adults in the US and usually develops in middle age. Gout is usually preceded by a period in which the uric acid levels in the blood are high. It is related to lifestyle factors, such as eating red meat and drinking excessive amounts of alcohol.

Risk factors

Genetics and gender are the main risk factors. The frequency of gout increases with age. Some of the uric acid that contributes to gout comes from a high intake of purines, essential molecules found in lentils, dried beans, sardines, shellfish, and organ meats. Most of the uric acid comes from within the body when purines and proteins are broken down.

■ **GENETIC** Many people with gout have an inherited tendency for their uric acid levels to be high.

■ **GENDER** Gout is about three times more common in men than in women. Gout rarely affects women before they reach menopause.

Q&A

Does everyone with high uric acid levels have gout?

No. And curiously, many patients who experience an acute attack of gout do not have raised uric acid levels. Nevertheless, it is true to say that the higher the uric acid levels, the more likely the chance of an attack of gout.

■ **MEDICAL TREATMENT** Uric acid levels may be raised either from cancer treatment, which causes cells to be broken down and purines to be released from DNA, or as a side-effect of thiazide diuretics, such as hydrochlorothiazide, which is used to treat high blood pressure.

What happens?

Gout can be triggered by illness, surgery, trauma, or a metabolic disturbance. Acute gout causes agony. There is a sudden onset of pain in a single joint, which is hot, red, and very tender to the touch. Some people have recurrent episodes; in others, gout is like rheumatoid arthritis, becoming chronic and destructive.

Uric acid is normally excreted in urine. When the balance between the amount produced and the amount excreted is upset, uric acid levels rise. When these are too high, crystals form and collect in the white cells in joints and other tissues. This can cause an acute arthritis with intense local pain.

Gout affects the joints, particularly in the big toe, where it can be very painful. In fact, in an acute attack, gout can be the most painful arthritis of all.

In gout, high levels of uric acid in the blood cause crystals of uric acid to accumulate in the synovial fluid and joint capsule of one or more joints. In an attack of gout, which may come without warning, the pain can be unbearable. The affected joint turns red with inflammation and swells up.

Gout most commonly and traditionally targets the joint at the base of the big toe where the pain is also the most excruciating. Others joints that can be affected include the elbows, knees, ankles, wrists, and hands.

The sharp, needlelike crystals also accumulate in other parts of the body—for example, under the skin where the white deposits are known as tophi. These tophi are usually found on the earlobes, but they can occur at many sites, including the soft tissues of the hands and feet. Crystals may also accumulate in the kidneys, where they form kidney stones and can cause renal failure.

In some people, the symptoms of pseudogout are very similar to those in rheumatoid arthritis and osteoarthritis.

Pseudogout

Like gout, acute arthritis can be caused when crystals of calcium pyrophosphate dihydrate are deposited in joints, particularly the knee and less often the big toe. This is known as pseudogout because of its similarity to gout.

Pseudogout affects more men than women when compared with gout, but it usually occurs later in life. It may also run in families. In some people, the symptoms of pseudogout are very similar to those in rheumatoid arthritis and osteoarthritis.

The exact source of the crystals and why they cause acute arthritis are unknown. There may be a link with abnormal connective tissue or cartilage, or with other disorders, such as an underactive thyroid gland, excess iron storage, an overactive parathyroid gland, and other causes of excess calcium in the blood. Episodes of pseudogout can follow surgery, metabolic disturbances, or an injury to a joint.

Crystals may collect in the cartilage around joints, especially in elderly people, without causing symptoms. Many elderly people with osteoarthritis can develop pseudogout when the crystals interact with their condition.

Q&A

Can tuberculosis cause arthritis?

Yes. Chronic infections such as tuberculosis can cause arthritis. About 1 percent of people with tuberculosis develop an associated arthritis. It particularly involves the spine, hips, knees, wrists, or ankles. often starting slowly and usually involving just one joint. Symptoms include a low-grade fever, increased sweating, fever at night, reduced joint mobility, and some swelling and tenderness of the joints.

Arthritis and infection

Many important but relatively uncommon forms of arthritis are due to infections with viruses, bacteria, or fungi. They can occur by themselves or sometimes, in the case of infective arthritis due to bacteria, can complicate a pre-existing inflammatory arthritis. They vary in their appearance and in the course they take.

Many forms of viral illness can cause an arthritis. This is usually of minor relevance, and aches and pains occur against a background of feeling generally unwell. A viral arthritis tends to affect many joints and involves joint pain rather than inflammation, with characteristic pain and stiffness. It often occurs in the later stages of a viral illness and may come with a mild fever.

Acute bacterial infection tends to cause arthritis in one or a few joints, which become inflamed and are hot, swollen, and red. There is usually a fever, too. Rarely, a severe sudden septic arthritis can affect a joint, with a high fever and severe ill-health. People with a preexisting arthritis are more likely to develop it.

Reactive arthritis

This inflammatory arthritis develops after a bacterial infection. It can be accompanied by rashes on the hands or feet, diarrhea, conjunctivitis, mouth ulcers, and inflammation of the genital tract, which produces a discharge from the vagina or penis.

Reactive arthritis usually lasts for 6 months or less and rarely has any long-term consequences. About 1 percent of people with an episode of infective diarrhea or a sexually acquired infection develop reactive arthritis.

Lyme disease

This disease was first identified in people from Old Lyme, Connecticut. Initial symptoms of Lyme disease, which is caused by a bacterium (see above), include fever, fatigue, muscle pain, and a rash. After some months, over half of infected people may develop arthritis, mainly in the large joints, especially the knees.

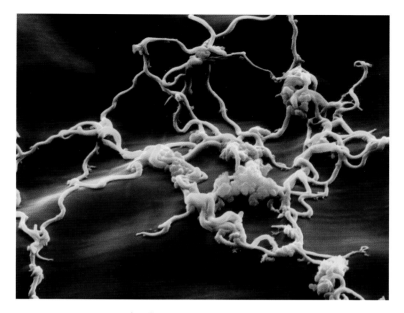

BORRELIA BURGDORFERI
The bacterium *Borrelia burgdorferi* (colored yellow above) causes Lyme disease in humans and is transmitted through a bite from an infected tick.

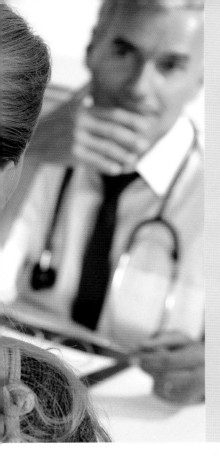

Related conditions

Many conditions involving joint pain or inflammation of soft tissues and other areas of the body may be related to arthritis. Other disorders, such as vasculitis and carpal tunnel syndrome, may accompany the different types of arthritis. If you have arthritis, you may be at a slightly increased risk of developing such disorders, but they are not an inevitable progression; any of them can also affect people who do not have arthritis, and some are rare. You should always consult your physician to obtain the correct diagnosis and treatment if you experience any of the symptoms described here.

Lupus has no cure but drugs can do much to relieve the symptoms and control the progression of the disease.

Lupus (SLE)

Systemic lupus erythematosus (SLE), or lupus for short, is a disease that causes inflammation in many parts of the body. The areas affected may include the joints, skin, and the tissues of the lungs, heart, and kidneys. The nervous system is sometimes involved, too. However, lupus rarely causes joint damage.

Lupus is a disorder of the immune system. It is not known what triggers the disease but viral infections, stress, and hormone imbalances may be involved. Certain drugs can occasionally cause side effects that resemble the symptoms of lupus. The disease is far more common in women than in men and is also more likely to occur in African-American and Asian women. Women with lupus should consult their physician if they are thinking of having a baby. Lupus is comparatively rare in children and does not usually develop in adults after the age of 50 unless it is due to a medication.

Symptoms and treatment

Lupus symptoms can vary considerably from one person to the next. The first symptoms are often aching and pain in the joints, particularly in the hands and feet. Another major symptom is a red skin rash, which typically spreads across the nose and cheeks but can appear elsewhere on the body (see below). Depression and a feeling of general fatigue are common.

Some people develop persistent mouth ulcers and experience hair loss. Inflammation of the lining of the heart and lungs can cause chest pain and shortness of breath. If the kidneys are affected, serious complications may arise, such as high blood pressure and kidney failure, but these are rare.

Lupus is highly variable. Many people are affected mildly while others may have severe symptoms that intermittently flare up and then subside for long periods. Permanent improvement is very rare. Lupus has no cure but drugs (see p.81) can do much to relieve the symptoms and control the progression of the disease.

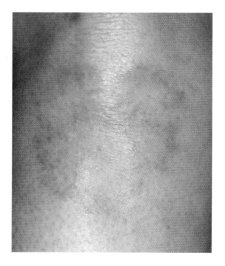

Fibromyalgia

The term fibromyalgia describes a collection of symptoms, the most important of which is persistent pain in many areas of the body. Fibromyalgia affects the muscles and other connective tissues, such as tendons and ligaments, and is not a joint disorder as such.

The cause of fibromyalgia is not known, but it may be linked to stress, anxiety, or depression. About 90 percent of people with fibromyalgia are women over the age of 40. Although this disorder may persist for many months or years, it does not cause damage to muscles or joints and will not lead to the development of arthritis or make existing arthritis worse.

Symptoms and treatment

The pain may occur anywhere, often on both sides of the body at once, and is usually experienced as widespread aching and stiffness. Typically, several small sites in particular areas—the base of the skull, around the shoulderblades or breastbone—are painful when pressed. Physicians use the number and distribution of these "tender points" to diagnose fibromyalgia (see p.28).

LUPUS SKIN RASH
A blotchy red rash on the skin is a common feature of lupus. The skin rashes tend to become worse if they are exposed to sunlight or ultraviolet radiation. In some instances, sunlight may even act as a trigger and cause the disease to flare up.

Poor posture can contribute to back pain, so you should check that you are not putting strain on soft tissues by sitting incorrectly at your desk or while driving.

Around 90 percent of people with fibromyalgia are affected by severe fatigue and have problems with sleeping. Other symptoms include headaches, irregular bowel movements that alternate between diarrhea and constipation (irritable bowel syndrome), and frequent need to urinate.

Fibromyalgia can be difficult to treat, although the symptoms may be eased in various ways. For example, analgesics may bring some relief and your physician may prescribe low-dose antidepressants to improve disturbed sleep. Self-help measures, such as low-impact exercise and applying gentle heat to painful areas, may also help.

Lower back pain

Lower back pain is one of the most common health complaints in adults. It can have many causes but is most frequently the result of a minor injury to the soft tissues of the back.

Symptoms and treatment

An acute pain in the lower back that develops suddenly is often due to a physical activity, such as lifting a heavy weight, that puts excessive strain on muscles or tendons. An injury of this type can cause a sharp pain in one specific place or a more widespread, dull aching, as well as stiffness when you bend down.

THE TENDER POINTS OF FIBROMYALGIA

Fibromyalgia can be difficult to diagnose so physicians rely on the presence of tender points, located in 9 symmetrical pairs, at particular sites around the body. Although this technique is not foolproof because tenderness can vary from day to day, fibromyalgia may be confirmed if 11 of the 18 points are tender when pressed. The pairs of tender points can be found in the following locations: at the base of the skull, at the base of the neck, on top of the shoulders, on the inside edge of the shoulderblades, below the elbows, at the top of the breastbone, at the low back, at the top of the outer thighs, and on the fat pad just above the inside of the knees.

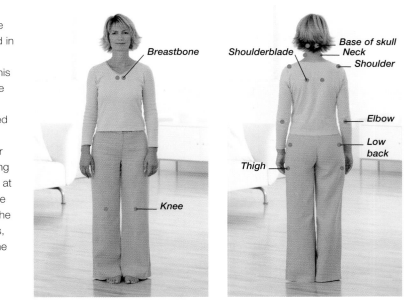

Breastbone

Shoulderblade — Base of skull
Neck
Shoulder

Elbow

Low back

Thigh

Knee

Poor posture is a more gradual way of contributing to back pain, so you should check that you are not putting strain on soft tissues by sitting incorrectly at your desk or while driving (see p.178.)

Another cause of back pain is a condition known commonly as a "slipped disk," in which one of the shock-absorbing pads of cartilage between two vertebrae is displaced (prolapsed) or damaged. If the disk presses against one of the nerves in the spine, you may experience severe pain, as well as numbness and tingling in one leg. Persistent lower back pain is frequently related to some types of arthritis, such as osteoarthritis or ankylosing spondylitis, which affect the joints of the spine.

Back pain due to minor tissue damage usually clears up within about 2 weeks. Your physician may suggest that you take analgesics and you could try self-help measures, such as applying a heat pad or an ice pack to your back, to ease the symptoms. Bed rest may help if you are in severe pain, but not for more than a day or two.

Localized soft-tissue disorders

The pain and inflammation in the following common conditions is confined to the soft tissues around specific joints.

INCIDENCE OF BACK PAIN

Back pain seems to strike when you are least expecting it or when a relatively minor action triggers a disproportionately painful episode. Statistics show that back problems are most likely to trouble you between the ages of 30 and 50, when the disks between your vertebrae are at their most vulnerable.

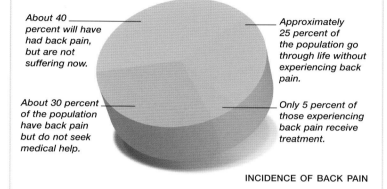

About 40 percent will have had back pain, but are not suffering now.

Approximately 25 percent of the population go through life without experiencing back pain.

About 30 percent of the population have back pain but do not seek medical help.

Only 5 percent of those experiencing back pain receive treatment.

INCIDENCE OF BACK PAIN

Bursitis

Joints are cushioned by fluid-filled sacs called bursae, which help reduce friction. In bursitis, a bursa becomes inflamed and tender, making the joint stiff and painful to move. The most common sites of bursitis are the knee, elbow, and shoulder. Persistently repeated movement or pressure are the usual causes; more rarely, it may be caused by an infection. Inflammatory disorders such as arthritis and gout can make you more susceptible to bursitis.

Resting the joint, applying ice packs, and anti-inflammatory drugs often relieve the symptoms. If the bursitis recurs or remains troublesome, your physician may suggest draining the bursa.

PRACTICAL TIPS

LOWER BACK PAIN

If you suddenly have an acute attack of pain in your lower back:

● Stay calm and don't panic. Just relax and breathe deeply.

● Keep your spine straight to take the weight off the disks of cartilage in your spine. Lie down or sit, whichever is the most comfortable, and rest.

● Contact your physician if the pain does not ease up.

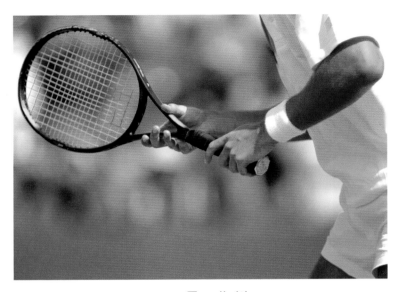

TENNIS ELBOW
Tennis elbow occurs when a tendon becomes inflamed and painful at the point where it is attached to a bone in the elbow.

Tendinitis

Tendinitis is the inflammation of a tendon, one of the tough, flexible cords that attach muscle to bone or muscle to muscle. It is often caused by injury or overstrain and occasionally by arthritis. In rare cases, the inflammation is due to an infection. In tendinitis, the synovium (the sheath of tissue surrounding the tendon) often becomes inflamed at the same time; this accompanying disorder is known as tenosynovitis.

Tendinitis and tenosynovitis cause pain and stiffness around a joint; the area may be swollen, red, and warm to touch. Tendons in the shoulder, elbow, knee, and heel are most likely to be affected. If you have rheumatoid arthritis, you may develop tenosynovitis in your fingers. Your physician may prescribe drugs to reduce the pain and inflammation.

Tennis elbow

Despite the name of the condition, in which the outer part of the elbow is inflamed and painful, it is not necessarily the result of playing tennis. Tennis elbow most often occurs when strenuous repetitive movements, such as those used in heavy manual work, cause tiny tears in the tendon. Tennis elbow may also be caused by a direct blow to the arm or may be a complication of arthritis.

Symptoms include pain and tenderness around the bony point of the elbow on the outside as well as stiffness. The pain is caused by damage to the tendon that attaches the muscles of the forearm to the upper arm bone (humerus). If you continue to overuse the arm, you may cause further damage to the tendon, and the pain and stiffness may gradually get worse.

For mild tennis elbow you can rest the arm, apply ice packs to the painful area, and take anti-inflammatory drugs. For more severe damage, your physician may suggest physical therapy, which includes gentle stretching exercises and possibly ultrasound treatment. If the condition does not improve within a few weeks, your physician may inject a corticosteroid into your elbow.

Plantar fasciitis

This painful foot disorder is the inflammation of the plantar fascia on the sole of the foot. Plantar fasciitis is usually the result of an injury. Older people are prone to this disorder because the tissues in their feet have lost some of their elasticity and their heels are not well cushioned to absorb shock. Plantar fasciitis also sometimes develops in people who gain weight suddenly, which can put extra strain on the load-bearing capacity of the feet.

The pain of plantar fasciitis, which may be a severe, stabbing sensation, is felt under the bottom of the heel (see below), especially when you first stand up in the morning. Sitting down may bring temporary relief, but the pain tends to return when you stand or walk for any length of time.

Your physician may suggest drugs that will reduce the inflammation. Wearing an arch support in your shoe and doing gentle stretching exercises may also help.

Sjögren's syndrome

This condition is an immune system disorder in which the tissues of lubricating glands, especially the glands that produce tears and saliva, are inflamed. The eyes become very dry and feel gritty; a lack of saliva in the mouth often causes difficulty swallowing. In women, the glands that moisten the vagina may also be affected. Occasionally, the joints are inflamed, causing symptoms similar to those of rheumatoid arthritis. Sjögren's syndrome is far more common in women than in men, and is most likely to develop in middle age.

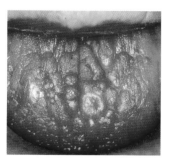

DRY TONGUE
In Sjögrens syndrome, the tongue dries out as the salivary glands stop producing saliva and start to waste away.

PAIN IN THE HEEL

Along the sole of each foot, stretching from the heel to the ball, there is a band of tough fibrous tissue called the plantar fascia. This tissue contributes to the shape of the arch of your foot and, at the same time, gives it support. Every day, it is subject to constant stresses as you walk or run or bend your foot in any way. Plantar fasciitis occurs when an area of the plantar fascia becomes inflamed where it attaches to the calcaneus bone of the heel.

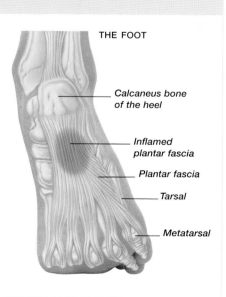

THE FOOT

Calcaneus bone of the heel

Inflamed plantar fascia

Plantar fascia

Tarsal

Metatarsal

Without treatment, carpal tunnel syndrome may eventually lead to permanent numbness in the hand, wasting of muscles, and a weakened grip.

There is no cure for the disorder but symptoms can be relieved with treatments such as artificial tears for dry eyes and, in severe cases, drugs to reduce inflammation.

Scleroderma

In scleroderma (the term means "hard skin"), the connective tissues that support and join together the various parts of the body become hard and thick. Believed to be an immune system abnormality, the disease most commonly affects the skin and joints, although internal organs may also be damaged.

Early symptoms include Raynaud's phenomenon, in which the fingers become cold, white, and swollen. Finger joints may be stiff and painful to move. Thickening of the skin sometimes develops over wide areas of the body and the skin may feel tight. Widespread scleroderma often

affects the esophagus (the tube that conveys food from the mouth to the stomach), stiffening the tissues, and causing difficulty swallowing as well as digestive problems. In severe cases, the tissue damage spreads to the lungs, heart, and kidneys, impairing their function and causing long-term complications.

Scleroderma cannot be cured although treatment with drugs can slow down its progression.

Accompanying conditions

A number of potentially serious conditions, such as carpal tunnel syndrome, polymyositis, vasculitis, and osteoporosis, may accompany some of the types of arthritis. However, this link with arthritis is not inevitable. At the same time, people who do not have arthritis may develop the conditions.

Carpal tunnel syndrome

In this condition, the main nerve to the hand is compressed as it passes through the wrist, causing numbness and tingling in the hand (see opposite). Pain may be felt in the wrist and up the forearm, too.

The cause of carpal tunnel syndrome is not always obvious, but it is sometimes linked to repetitive hand movements that cause swelling of the soft tissues within the carpal tunnel (see

REPETITIVE STRAIN
People who spend hours in front of a computer put the joints of their wrists and fingers under repeated strain and may develop carpal tunnel syndrome.

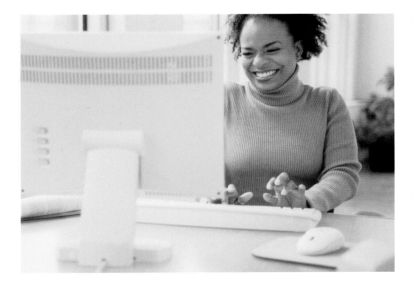

right). Damage to the joints of the wrist, due to injury or arthritis, may also cause narrowing of the carpal tunnel.

Many people find that their symptoms are often most severe at night or when they wake in the morning. Without treatment, carpal tunnel syndrome may eventually lead to permanent numbness in the hand, wasting of muscles, and a weakened grip.

Wearing a wrist splint or practicing a yoga pose called namaste (see right) may bring relief. If symptoms are particularly bad, your physician may prescribe anti-inflammatory drugs. In some cases, surgery may relieve pressure on the median nerve.

Polymyositis and dermatomyositis

These two rare disorders are types of soft-tissue inflammation that may develop at the same time. Both occur more commonly in children than in adults.

In polymyositis, the muscles are affected, especially around the pelvis and in the shoulders, causing weakness and pain. People with this condition may have difficulty raising their hands above their heads, getting up from a chair, or climbing stairs. If the condition worsens, the muscles of the throat, chest, and heart may also become damaged. This may then cause difficulty swallowing and shortness of breath.

CARPAL TUNNEL SYNDROME

The carpal tunnel is the gap between the wrist bones (carpals). The median nerve passes through the tunnel, underneath a band of ligament, and branches into nerves that serve the fingers and the thumb. These nerves control some of the muscles of the hand. In carpal tunnel syndrome, pressure on the median nerve causes numbness and tingling, particularly in the first and middle fingers and the thumb.

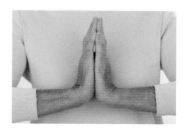

NAMASTE YOGA POSE
A yoga pose callled namaste can bring relief to the pain of carpal tunnel syndrome. The palms are held together in front of the chest, with the elbows pointing out to the sides.

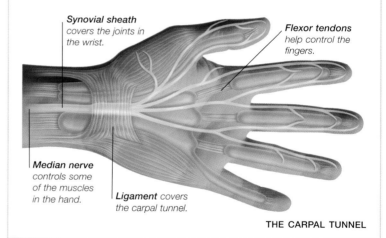

Synovial sheath covers the joints in the wrist.

Flexor tendons help control the fingers.

Median nerve controls some of the muscles in the hand.

Ligament covers the carpal tunnel.

THE CARPAL TUNNEL

In dermatomyositis, a rash occurs, most often appearing on the face and the backs of the hands. Typically, the eyelids become swollen and turn a reddish purple. In children, severe dermatomyositis may also cause skin ulcers.

There is no cure for polymyositis and dermatomyositis, but your physician may prescribe drug treatment to reduce inflammation and improve the symptoms.

VASCULITIS

Inflammation of the body's blood vessels, known by the general term of vasculitis, may accompany inflammatory arthritis. One form of vasculitis is giant cell arteritis (also called Horton's disease), which is caused by a response of the immune system. Giant cell arteritis usually affects the cranial and temporal arteries of the head in the elderly, causing headaches.

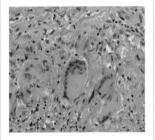

GIANT CELL ARTERITIS
The most characteristic feature of the condition is the presence of giant cells—one such cell can be seen at the center of the light micrograph.

However, in the majority of affected children who are affected, the disorders usually disappear completely within about two years. On the other hand, adults who are affected are likely to need long-term treatment.

Polymyalgia rheumatica

In this disorder, pain and stiffness affect many muscles, mainly in the neck, shoulders, and around the hips and thighs. The symptoms, which may develop gradually but can also sometimes appear very rapidly, may include fever, night sweats, general fatigue and weakness, and depression. In some people, polymyalgia rheumatica is associated with giant cell arteritis (see left and below).

The cause of the disorder is not known. Women are more likely to be affected than men and the disorder is rare in people under the age of 50. Treatment is usually with drugs to relieve pain and reduce inflammation.

Blood vessel disorders

Inflammation of the blood vessels, known as vasculitis, sometimes occurs in conjunction with other inflammatory disorders, such as rheumatoid arthritis, although the condition can also develop in people with no previous health problems. Vasculitis can affect all types of blood vessels: arteries, veins, and capillaries. Two forms of vasculitis are described below.

■ **WEGENER'S GRANULOMATOSIS** The typical symptom is inflammation of the blood vessels that supply the tissues of the nasal passages, lungs, and kidneys. As the disease progresses, it causes abnormal groups of cells called granulomas to form and eventually replace healthy tissues.

Symptoms often first appear in the respiratory tract and can include nosebleeds, inflamed sinuses, coughing up of phlegm that is sometimes bloodstained, and shortness of breath.

These symptoms may be accompanied by fever, aches and pains, and fatigue. Sometimes the middle ear is inflamed. If it affects the kidneys it may prevent the normal filtering of waste products from the blood. Long-term drug treatment may be needed to prevent complications from arising.

■ **GIANT CELL ARTERITIS** Also known as temporal arteritis, this affects the arteries in the head and neck, most commonly the temporal arteries, which lie just beneath the skin of the temples. The name of the condition comes from the abnormally large cells that develop in the blood vessel walls (see left).

The first symptom is usually a headache, sometimes severe, on one or both sides of the head. Affected arteries may be swollen and the scalp tender. The disorder sometimes occurs at the same time as polymyalgia rheumatica.

Prompt treatment of giant cell arteritis is required because complications can include permanent blindness in one or both eyes. Drugs to reduce the inflammation are usually effective, although some people need to take medication for several years to control the condition.

Osteoporosis

This condition is very different from arthritis because the bones lose their density, becoming weakened and brittle. However, it can be an added complication for people who already have arthritis.

Bone structure is maintained by a lifelong process that creates bone cells (osteoblasts) and breaks them down. As people age, bone cells are broken down faster than they are replaced and bone becomes lighter and more porous.

Osteoporosis affects everyone to some extent with age and as the production of sex hormones, essential for bone maintenance, starts to decline. Women are especially susceptible once they reach menopause because their levels of estrogen fall rapidly as their ovaries cease production (see p.192).

Just as exercise can increase bone strength, people who remain bedridden or inactive for long periods because of illness can lose bone mass very quickly. Some long-term drug treatments, such as those used in arthritis, can also speed up the loss of bone density.

Osteoporosis does not in itself cause pain, but it does increase the likelihood of fractures. In fact, the first sign of weakened bones is usually a fracture, often following a comparatively minor fall. In older people, common sites of fracture are the wrist or hip.

If osteoporosis affects the spine, the back may become rounded with a noticeable loss of height. When the vertebrae become seriously weakened, a fracture of one or more of them may occur spontaneously, which may cause severe back pain.

Once you have lost bone mass it can no longer be replaced with the oral drugs currently available. Drugs may be recommended to slow further progress of osteoporosis and to minimize the risk of fractures. There are also preventive measures you can take to protect yourself against further bone loss (see p.194).

When treatment for osteoporosis is needed, bisphosphonate drugs (including alendronate, residronate, and ibandronate) are usually prescribed. These may cause stomach problems. Calcitonin and raloxifene are less frequently used. Teriparatide, derived from human parathyroid hormone and given as a daily injection for 2 years, is the only therapy that can build new bone.

As people age, bone is broken down faster than it is replaced and the skeleton becomes lighter and more porous.

HIGH-IMPACT EXERCISE
Building up the strength of your bones with high-impact exercise can help prevent osteoporosis— and it can also be enjoyable.

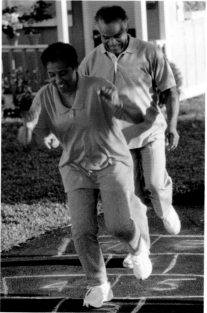

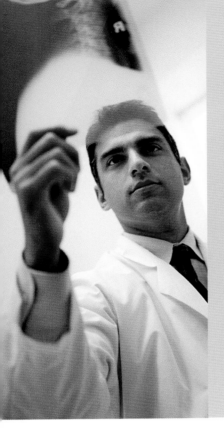

Symptoms and diagnosis

For most people with arthritis, pain is the most immediate predominant symptom. Other symptoms, such as inflammation and stiffness, are due either to the disease itself or to its consequences. When a rheumatologist looks at all your symptoms together, a particular pattern emerges that will help narrow down and identify the type of arthritis that is affecting you. Such diagnoses are often determined and confirmed by a range of techniques—from X–rays to blood tests—at the rheumatologist's disposal.

The impact of arthritis is to make people less able to live normally and more likely to be disabled.

Recognizing arthritis

Symptoms vary enormously from person to person, depending on both the type of arthritis and its extent and severity. Symptoms are also greatly influenced by personal factors unique to the individual. The symptoms key to recognizing arthritis are pain, inflammation, stiffness, loss of function, joint damage, and fatigue.

Pain
The dominant symptom in all types of arthritis, and indeed in every type of musculoskeletal disease, is pain. Inflamed joints are painful both at rest and when they are moved. People with arthritis usually seek medical advice because they want relief from the pain in their joints.

The subjective sensation of pain in arthritis is very personal. It affects different people in different ways. The exact description of the nature of the pain does not help in the diagnosis of the condition.

Unlike many forms of pain, the pain of arthritis is chronic, which means that it is present most of the time and lasts for long periods. People with long-term pain experience all sorts of other effects, such as depression.

In arthritis, pain is normally associated with joint tenderness: when a joint is pressed it hurts. The more active the arthritis, the more joints are tender. The number of tender joints is one measure of the severity of arthritis.

Inflammation and swelling

A joint that is inflamed becomes swollen. Either the lining of the joint swells (synovitis) or the synovial fluid increases in volume (an effusion). The number of swollen joints is a good indication of the severity of the arthritis.

Inflammation in a joint is no different from inflammation elsewhere in the body. It is an active process: inflammatory cells (mainly white cells) and more blood enter into the joint, while many inflammatory molecules, such as small proteins (peptides), are released into the soft tissues around the joint. The increased blood flow makes the joint swell and feel warm. The inflammatory materials cause fluid to collect in and around the joint, which adds to the swelling.

Stiffness

Inflamed joints can feel stiff first thing in the morning. How long it lasts is important: an hour or more is suggestive of inflammatory arthritis. Defining morning stiffness is hard, although people with arthritis describe it as an ache combined with difficulty moving.

Stiffness following exercise is usually a feature of osteoarthritis; it is a sign that the joints are starting to fail. People feel stiff when they rest, such as sitting down after a walk or relaxing in the evening. The joints are sometimes said to "gel," a term reminiscent of how gelatine sets— a gradual process of firming up.

Loss of function

When joints are painful, swollen, and stiff they start to lose their function: they do not work well or move properly. As a result,

IDENTIFYING SYMPTOMS

Pain, inflammation, swelling, and stiffness are the four symptoms that doctors look for when trying to identify arthritis. Sometimes, these symptoms are accompanied by other features, such as loss of function and a sensation of unbearable fatigue, or general symptoms that affect the body as a whole.

SYMPTOMS	WHAT THEY MEAN
Pain	Pain in a joint or joints may be mild, moderate, or severe, and is usually chronic. Joint pain is a symptom of all types of arthritis.
Inflammation	Inflammation is a symptom of the various types of inflammatory arthritis, as well as many instances of osteoarthritis.
Swelling	Either the lining of the joint swells or fluid flows into the joint. Usually indicates inflammatory arthritis.
Stiffness	Morning stiffness that lasts more than an hour usually indicates a form of inflammatory arthritis. Stiffness that follows exercise usually suggests osteoarthritis.

A complex and subtle issue is the way arthritis can change people's appearance and the way they look at themselves.

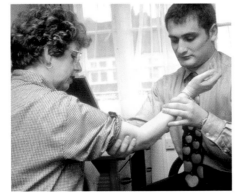

everyday tasks become hard to complete. Arthritis of the hands causes difficulty with cooking and eating. Arthritis of the knees and feet causes difficulty with walking. The overall impact of arthritis is to make people less able to live normal lives and more likely to become disabled.

The ways in which arthritis can affect an individual are relative and depend on many circumstances. For example, a previously fit person may be less disabled than an unfit person. Losing function is also subjective; what some people find an inconvenience to others represents a personal disaster. This does not merely mean that some people cope well with problems while others do not. It is more complicated than that. For example, a professional musician who plays the violin or piano would find arthritis of the hands far more of a problem than someone who spends his or her time talking to others without the need for physical performance.

Changes in self-perception

A complex and subtle issue is the way arthritis can change people's appearance and the way they look at themselves. How we look is of fundamental importance to us all. In the long-term, arthritis affects both self-image and actual appearance, with consequent changes in self-perception. While these are difficult to quantify, they change a person's quality of life rather than cause a distinct disability, and are important end results of arthritis.

Joint damage

Inflammation that persists can cause damage to an arthritic joint. Eventually, the damage becomes irreversible and the joints look distinctly different. The final common pathway of the damage is one of osteoarthritis and joint failure, but the early stages differ between the types of arthritis and the joints affected.

Damage to cartilage and bone is also accompanied by damage to tendons and soft tissues around joints. This may not be obvious at first, but later it can cause very typical abnormalities. For example, in rheumatoid arthritis tendon damage causes a number of specific changes in the fingers, such as the "swan-neck" deformity.

Fatigue

A marked feature of arthritis is a sensation of unbearable fatigue. It is closely related to pain and its effect on mood—possibly even causing depression, which is common in arthritis. The fatigue is due to poor sleep, weakened muscles, and a disease process that affects the whole body and mind.

General symptoms

Extensive joint inflammation—for example, in severe rheumatoid arthritis—may be accompanied by a low-grade fever, loss of weight, and a feeling of being generally unwell. This is because the illness affects the whole body.

Rashes are a feature in a few types of arthritis, such as psoriatic arthritis and lupus. However, in most people they are a relatively common side effect of treatment.

Diagnosing arthritis

After first assessing your personal circumstances and health status, your doctor can recommend blood tests and imaging techniques, such as X-rays, to help confirm —or discard—a diagnosis of a particular type of arthritis. If the diagnosis is still in question, however, a magnetic resonance imaging (MRI) scan may be ordered (see right).

History and examination

Your doctor will assess you by listening to your medical history and looking at what is wrong (the examination).

Your medical history has a number of features: the history of the arthritis itself; general problems; current and previous treatments; details of past diseases; the occurrence of arthritis in your relatives; and your work and social

---

MRI SCANNING

Examination of a joint, such as the knee, with a magnetic resonance imaging (MRI) scan can reveal the extent of osteoarthritis. A MRI scan literally takes an image of a slice of your body and reveals soft tissues that are not normally visible on X–rays. The MRI scan of a knee joint (below) belongs to a man who developed osteoarthritis at the unusually early age of 33. The scan shows the lower end of the thigh bone (femur) and the upper end of the shin bone (tibia). Due to osteoarthritis the bone tissue at the end of the thigh bone has become eroded and jagged. Cracks that have opened up at the end of both the bones will weaken the joint.

MRI SCANNER
A magnetic resonance imaging (MRI) scanner houses a large magnet that can make images of slices of your body. You need to lie very still on a narrow table inside a tunnel. If you are concerned about feeling claustrophobic, make sure your doctor knows so that you can be given a sedative.

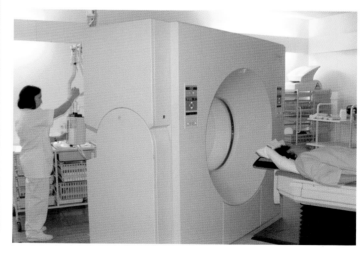

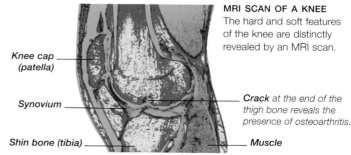

Knee cap (patella)

Synovium

Shin bone (tibia)

MRI SCAN OF A KNEE
The hard and soft features of the knee are distinctly revealed by an MRI scan.

Crack at the end of the thigh bone reveals the presence of osteoarthritis.

Muscle

ARTHROSCOPY AND BIOPSY

Fiberoptic arthroscopes, which are small and flexible, can be used to look inside large joints, such as the knee, and small joints, such as the wrist. For example, arthroscopy of the knee can distinguish between problems due to meniscus damage (torn knee cartilage) and problems resulting from arthritis. Arthroscopes can also be used to obtain a biopsy of the synovial tissue of some joints to check for infections, crystals, and abnormal cells.

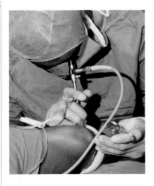

ARTHROSCOPY
With a fiberoptic arthroscope, a surgeon can examine a joint very thoroughly and precisely identify a problem.

situation. The physical examination will focus on your muscles and joints in particular.

To the uninitiated it might seem that clinicians ask a whole series of questions, complete a full examination, and then reach a conclusion. In practice, the situation is quite different. If an expert clinician does not have a fairly good idea of the likely diagnosis during the first visit, it will probably take further testing to reach a diagnosis.

Most of your history is taken down as a way of ensuring that there is sufficient information to confirm first suspicions about the diagnosis and gaining information about you to recommend the most appropriate treatment.

The physical examination helps the physician make a diagnosis, and also helps in the evaluation of disease severity and the specific joints affected. It may reveal abnormalities that the patient did not notice, such as tophi.

X–rays
Plain radiographs (X–rays) are the classic method of imaging joints. They demonstrate joint damage and can provide a readily available assessment of its severity and progression. They can show localized bone loss, which in essence means the presence of erosions—a characteristic of rheumatoid arthritis. X–rays also show where there are bone spurs,

in particular the presence of osteophytes in osteoarthritis and also show loss of joint space. X–rays can help a doctor decide whether or not joint replacement surgery might be needed in a patient with disabling pain.

Other imaging techniques
There are a number of other ways of scanning the joints, such as computerized tomography (CT), magnetic resonance imaging (MRI), isotope bone scans, ultrasound, and dual energy X–ray absortiometry (DXA). Some, particularly MRI and ultrasound, can show inflammation and soft-tissue swelling. Others, especially DXA, show the presence of osteoporosis (see p.35).

Many techniques provide improved imaging of bones and joints compared to X–rays. More technically demanding and more expensive than routine radiology, they are, at present, used only in a minority of cases.

Blood tests
Analysis of the blood can help confirm a diagnosis or indicate the severity of the disease. The tests are never diagnostic in their own right. They are often used to assess the safety and effectiveness of treatment too.

■ **ASSESSING THE BODY'S RESPONSE** Blood tests can assess the normal way in which the body responds to a damaging situation, such as an infection. In some forms of arthritis, especially rheumatoid arthritis, the response is switched on when it should not be. This response can be detected when the erythrocyte sedimentation rate (ESR) increases (see right).

■ **TESTING FOR MARKERS** Blood tests can look for specific chemicals that are markers of arthritis. The most common test of this type measures uric acid levels in the blood. Uric acid levels are usually, but not necessarily, raised in people with gout. However, it is also true that in most individuals who have a high uric acid level there is no evidence of gout. In addition, in an acute attack of gout, serum uric acid levels may be normal.

■ **TESTING FOR AUTOANTIBODIES** Blood tests can identify specific auto-antibodies, such as rheumatoid factor (see below). Autoantibodies

are antibodies that react with specific proteins in your own body. They are thought to be the by-products of a disturbed immune system, which is a common feature in rheumatoid arthritis and some connective tissue diseases.

However, there is a paradox. The presence of autoantibodies does not mean that one or other of these diseases is present; indeed, most people with an autoantibody do not have arthritis. In addition, their absence does not rule out any disease. Nevertheless, most people who have an inflammatory arthritis (such as rheumatoid arthritis) or a connective tissue disease, such as lupus, will have a detectable level of an autoantibody in their blood. The higher the level of autoantibodies, the greater the chance of having severe disease.

■ **ANTINUCLEAR ANTIBODIES** Antinuclear antibodies react with components of the normal cell nucleus. They are characteristic of lupus, but also occur in most other connective tissue diseases, rheumatoid arthritis, and other generalized chronic inflammatory conditions. They are a family of different autoantibodies rather than a single and distinct autoantibody, and as a result they are very nonspecific. Nevertheless, it is usual for people with lupus to have some detectable antinuclear antibodies in their blood.

Q&A

What is rheumatoid factor?

Rheumatoid factor is the best known autoantibody. It is detected in about two-thirds of people with rheumatoid arthritis. It is an antibody that reacts with proteins called immunoglobulins that are part of the body's immune response. The higher the level of rheumatoid factor, the more severe the disease. Rheumatoid factor does not necessarily indicate rheumatoid arthritis because it can be associated with other diseases, too.

ERYTHROCYTE SEDIMENTATION

Red cells (erythrocytes) in the blood settle when left to stand; the erythrocyte sedimentation rate (ESR) test measures how fast. The faster they settle, the higher the ESR. It is measured in millimeters per hour. A normal ESR is less than 20. The ESR in active rheumatoid arthritis can be between 50 and 100. At the same time, there is a small fall in red cell numbers and changes in specific proteins in the blood. The most frequently measured protein is the quantitive C-reactive protein. Normally less than 5mg/liter in the blood, in active arthritis it can be 50–100mg/liter.

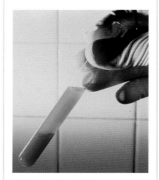

RED BLOOD CELLS

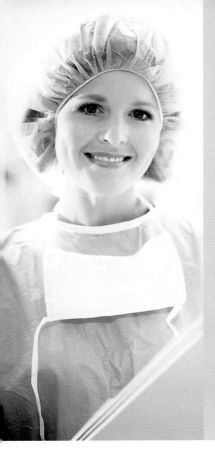

Looking after your arthritis

There is no need to feel helpless about a diagnosis of arthritis. Today, there are more treatment options available to you than ever before, from drugs and surgery to self-help measures and counseling. But no longer do you have to be a mere recipient of treatment. Increasingly, your input in helping manage your own arthritis will be welcomed and encouraged by many physicians and other health professionals who may be involved in both diagnosis and treatment.

Building up a working partnership with your physician will increase your confidence and help you feel in control of your arthritis.

Working with your healthcare professionals

If you have arthritis, you are likely to need regular health care on a long-term basis. Establishing a good relationship with your physician and other practitioners, such as physical therapists and nurses, can help reduce the stress and anxiety of coping with treatment and consultations.

Most importantly, mutual trust and understanding between you and your health professionals gives you the best chance of getting the treatment that is exactly right for you.

Two-way communication

Communication is the key to successful health care. As a patient, you can expect to receive the information your need from your physician. It is equally important that he or she receives information from you.

Physicians can learn a great deal about your condition from tests and physical examinations, but there are things they will not necessarily find out unless you tell them. Your personal knowledge of how arthritis—and its treatment—affects you is valuable to your physician. Don't hesitate to share your concerns and feel confident about speaking openly about your needs, symptoms, and feelings. Building a working partnership with your physician will increase your confidence and help you feel in control of your arthritis.

Making the most of your physician's appointment

Visiting the physician's office or a hospital appointment can be daunting, especially if you are newly diagnosed with arthritis. You may find it easier if you ask a friend or relative to accompany you to the appointment. Another person not only provides moral support if you are nervous, but can help you make sure that you ask the questions and get the answers you need.

Physicians have many responsibilities and most of them have only a short period of time in which to see individual patients, so make the best use of their time—and yours—by being well prepared for your appointment. Before you go, make a list of the important questions you want to ask or points you wish to discuss. Keep this list as concise as possible by focusing on the essentials.

Medical terminology can be confusing, so if you do not understand what your physician tells you, don't hesitate to ask him or her to repeat it or to explain things more simply. If you want more information, say so. Take a notepad with you to write down anything that you need to remember—it is easy to forget what has been said once you leave the physician's office. If you run out of time to discuss everything you want, schedule another appointment.

PRACTICAL TIPS

WHAT YOU CAN DO

● Keep a diary to monitor your progress and the effects of any treatment. It will provide a convenient record to discuss with your health professionals.

● If you are not satisfied with your health care, tell your physician—if you have a good patient-physician relationship, this will not cause offence.

● Don't be afraid to suggest alternative treatments to your physician, but be guided by his or her advice.

● When talking to your health professionals, be honest about how arthritis affects your personal life and emotional well-being.

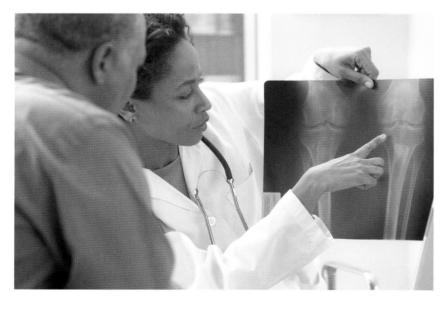

DISCUSSING YOUR ARTHRITIS
An appointment with your physician is the best time to discuss your arthritis and to communicate your thoughts and feelings about the condition.

PRACTICAL TIPS

SELF-HELP STRATEGIES

You may find that drugs or surgery alone do not control your arthritis. Regardless of whether you need extra medical help, the following self-help strategies will make a difference and almost certainly improve your quality of life overall. They may even bring some relief from symptoms such as pain and inflammation.

● Make changes to your lifestyle.

● Think positively about your arthritis.

● Participate in a sport (see p.64) or do exercise sequences (see p.158).

● Learn to cope with your stress (see p.152).

● Eat well (see p.50).

● Practice relaxation and meditation (see p.156).

● A complementary therapy (see pp.108–131) may also help you take control of your arthritis.

Getting the most from your treatment

Take an active role in your arthritis management plan by learning as much as you can about different treatment options and what you can expect from them. Being informed allows you to be more involved in decisions regarding your health care.

Management of arthritis differs from person to person, according to the severity of the condition and factors such as how individuals tolerate certain drugs. What suits one may not work as well with another—so make sure that your health professionals are aware of your personal needs and concerns. The more a physician knows about you and your lifestyle, the more precisely he or she can tailor treatment to your particular requirements.

Keep your physician up to date with aspects of your treatment that affect your quality of life. For example, your medication may be causing unacceptable side-effects or your exercise program may prove too strenuous. Discussing these problems as soon as they occur allows you and your physician to work together to prevent small problems from turning into major ones. You should also report the good news of any improvements. If you develop a new medical condition or a reaction to a medication in between office visits, call the physician to discuss the problem rather than waiting until your next appoinment.

Be a considerate patient

Your relationship with healthcare professionals will benefit if your expectations are reasonable. Always arrive on time for an appointment; if you have to cancel, tell the physician's office as soon as you can. If you are on refillable prescriptions, request a refill or get a new prescription before you run out of tablets.

Your treatment options

The treatment chosen will depend on a range of factors, including the type and severity of your arthritis, potential side-effects, and, of course, your own feelings and lifestyle concerns.

Drug treatment

A wide variety of drugs may be prescribed by physicians or bought over the counter at pharmacies. These include analgesics, non-steroidal anti-inflammatory drugs (NSAIDs), steroids, disease-modifying antirheumatic drugs, (DMARDs), and biologic agents (see pp.76–87)

Over-the-counter medicines

Many analgesics (see p.76) and NSAIDs (see p.78) are available over the counter, but in lower doses than those your physician would prescribe. All other drugs that are used to treat arthritis are available only on prescription. You should always read the package information carefully and make sure you take the correct dosage. Over-the-counter medicines can be dangerous if not taken properly.

Generic vs. brand drugs

All medicines have a generic name. Acetaminophen and ibuprofen are examples of generic names. Generic drugs are usually cheaper than brand names.

Brands and generics usually contain different buffers, additives, and fillers, but the active ingredients are the same. Strict laws ensure that both generic and brand-name drugs are equally effective and safe to use.

Q&A

Is it safe to buy drugs through the internet?

The Food and Drug Administration and organizations such as the American Medical Association and the Arthritis Foundation have warned against buying drugs through the internet. Although there are genuine online pharmacies, many have no regulations or controls so the drugs they offer may not be safe or of good quality, and vital patient information may be missing. Buy medicines only from regular pharmacies and on the advice of your physician.

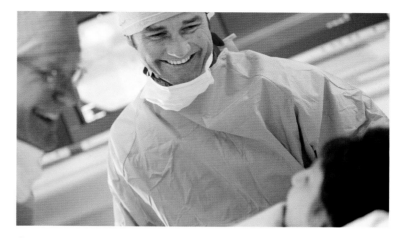

MEETING YOUR SURGEON
Before you have surgery to treat your arthritis you will have an opportunity to talk to the surgeon who will be performing the operation.

Surgery

When drugs cannot control your arthritis because of the extensive damage to the joints involved, your rheumatologist may suggest surgery (see pp.88–107). It may take some time to schedule an operation so don't delay making a decision.

Joint replacement, particularly of the hips, is common, although surgeons can also replace joints in the shoulders, knees, ankles, elbows, wrists, and fingers. They can also remove the lining in a joint, remove bone, and fuse joints to make them more stable.

Professional care

Many different health professionals may be involved in the diagnosis and treatment of your arthritis. Some you may see once only, others more than once or on an ongoing basis, depending on the type and severity of your arthritis.

Physicians

Your physician is your partner in caring for your arthritis. He or she can examine your joints and look for signs of swelling or reduced mobility. Your physician can refer you to a specialist in arthritis care (a rheumatologist) or to a nearby hospital for an array of tests.

Rheumatologists

Rheumatologists are specialists who have undergone 2 or 3 years of training in arthritis and other diseases that affect the joints, bones, and muscles beyond their general medical education. Some rheumatologists have their own offices; others are hospital-based. A rheumatologist can interpret your tests and may suggest further investigations. He or she will discuss your treatment and can prescribe drugs or refer you for surgery if that is required.

Children who are suspected of having arthritis (see p.182) may need to be referred to a pediatric rheumatologist. Alternatively, a regular rheumatologist may be able to help.

Orthopedic specialists

You may be referred to an orthopedist or to a surgeon who specializes in muscle and bone disorders. Orthopedic surgeons perform joint replacement surgery, back surgery, and arthroscopic surgery.

Physical therapists

A physical therapist is a specialist in physical treatments that help restore movement and function in the body. He or she may employ a wide range of different methods, from massage and manipulation to the use of heat and hydrotherapy. At the first session you will be asked about your condition and examined. A course of treatment, which may require further sessions, may be recommended.

Occupational therapists

If your arthritis causes practical problems at home or at work the best person to turn to for help is an occcupational therapist. They are usually based in a hospital or clinic. Ask your physician to refer you. (See also p.144.)

Nurses and nurse practitioners

Nurses at your health center or your physician's office, or at the hospital organize blood tests and provide advice on medication, among their many other roles. Nurse practitioners are highly experienced nurses who have extra training that allows them to take on certain roles traditionally carried out only by physicians.

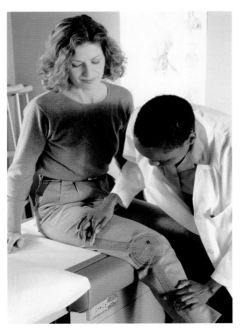

PHYSICAL THERAPY
Physical therapists may employ various techniques and physical treatments to help people with arthritis restore normal movement to their joints.

Dietitians and nutritionists

If you need to lose weight, your physician may refer you to a dietitian for advice on what foods are best for you to eat, and in what proportions. Dietitians must follow an established training program and be registered to practice. Nutritionists have a very similar role, but while they may also have undergone proper training they are not required to be registered.

Counseling

All physicians agree that pain is a complex and little-understood process and many people believe there is a strong link between the mind and body. Talking things through with a professional counselor may help you make a very real difference in your level of pain and discomfort.

You can ask your physician or rheumatologist to recommend a counselor who has had extensive experience in treating people with arthritis. If you consult a counselor privately, make sure he or she is either registered with an organization such as the American Association of Psychotherapists or is a licensed marriage and family counselor.

Support groups

These are a good way of keeping up to date on new treatments for arthritis, learning tips on coping with your pain and condition,

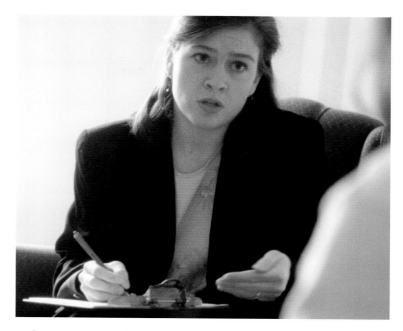

and getting in touch with others who share your experiences or problems.

Most support groups provide help lines or free Internet information. An example is the Arthritis Foundation (see Useful Addresses, p.217).

Pain clinics

Another solution to management of long-term pain are pain clinics. These clinics typically employ a wide variety of professionals, ranging from nurses and physicians, to complementary practitioners, including acupuncturists, and others who use drug injections, hydrotherapy, and other methods to control and relieve pain. Your physician will be able to locate the pain clinic closest to you.

COUNSELING
Healthcare professionals will provide you with all kinds of treatment, advice, and guidance that will help you look after yourself and manage your arthritis.

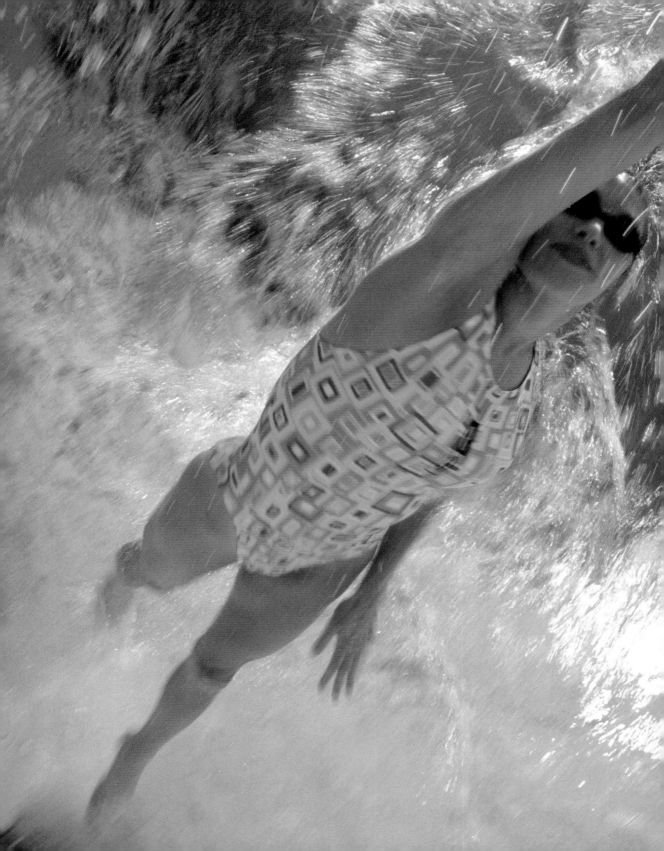

Food, drink, and physical activity

Eating a balanced diet and exercising regularly is good advice for everyone, but it is especially important if you have arthritis. These two crucial aspects of everyday life not only make you feel better but they also help you manage your weight.

While there is no evidence that specific foods can cure or cause arthritis, medical research suggests that some nutrients, such as omega-3 fatty acids, may be able to help relieve the symptoms. However, the best advice is to follow a diet that is rich in oily fish, fruit, vegetables, and low-fat dairy products, rather than relying on supplements or superfoods.

Regular physical activity and exercise can bring you many benefits. But you don't need to overdo it—just stay within your comfort zone. Your joints will become more mobile and flexible, while the adjacent muscles and other soft tissues remain healthy. Perhaps the best benefit of exercise is in keeping stiffness at bay and bring some welcome relief from pain.

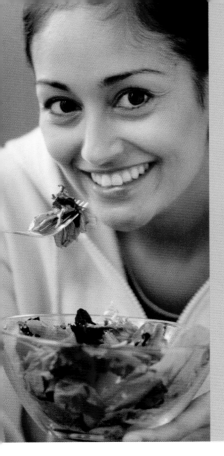

Eating to ease your arthritis

It is a popular belief that what you eat can relieve the inflammation and pain of arthritis. Some people are also convinced that certain foods can trigger their arthritis attacks. However, in most cases there is no firm medical evidence to confirm this. Your doctor may discourage you from emphasizing the links between food and arthritis, but there are good reasons for paying attention to your diet. As our understanding of arthritis progresses, it is becoming clear that what you eat may have potential benefits.

If you are getting the right nutrients you will maximize your chances of fighting disease.

Food and arthritis

People with arthritis need to eat the type of well-balanced diet that would be a healthy choice for anyone, regardless of his or her age or fitness. As a general guide, meals should include oily fish, low-fat or non-fat dairy products, lots of fresh fruits and vegetables, and only occasional greasy deep-fried foods and sugary treats. Meat-eaters can also have poultry and occasional red meat.

Many unsubstantiated claims have been made for the benefits of eliminating specific foods or food groups, or focusing on so-called "superfoods," to reduce pain and inflammation; regard these with extreme caution. Dietitians and physicians do not recommend such diets because they could possibly be detrimental to your general health. If you do want to try a special diet, always first consult a registered dietitian recommended by your physician.

What makes up a healthy diet?

Healthy eating entails choosing a variety of foods that will supply the energy (calories) your body needs to keep all its systems functioning normally. If you get the right nutrients you will maximize your body's ability to fight disease.

The five essential components of food are: carbohydrates, protein, fats, vitamins, and minerals. You need some of these components in larger quantities than others; the key to a healthy diet is getting the right balance.

Carbohydrates

Carbohydrates are our main source of energy. They are found mainly in starchy foods—such as bread, cereals, rice, pasta, and potatoes— and in sugar. Starchy foods also contain fiber and some nutrients essential to good health, including calcium, iron, and B vitamins. Sugar provides only calories and is of little nutritional value.

Starchy foods should make up about a third of what you eat. Whole-grain or wholewheat varieties of cereals, bread, rice, and pasta are the best options because they contain more fiber than the white varieties. It is fiber that keeps you feeling fuller for longer—it also helps keep your bowels functioning effectively.

Try to include starchy foods in each main meal. For example, start the day with a whole-grain cereal or freshly prepared hot oatmeal. (Some packet varieties of oatmeal may be full of sugar. If you need a sweetener, add some dried fruit or a banana instead.)

At lunch you could have a sandwich made with whole-grain bread, pita, or chapatti. For your evening meal you could include whole-grain bread, sweet potatoes, whole-grain pasta, or brown rice.

MYTH OR TRUTH?

MYTH

Food sensitivities play a major role provoking the symptoms of arthritis.

TRUTH

Most inflammation is not caused by sensitivity to one particular food, although some people do find that certain foods worsen their symptoms. It is better to follow a diet that is rich in the foods that are good for your health and may help lessen inflammation, rather than to focus on potential dietary culprits. Eliminating entire food groups can deprive your body of important nutrients.

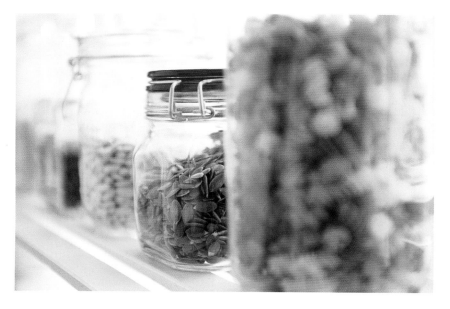

PASTA, LEGUMES, AND GRAINS
The wide variety of pasta, legumes, and grains provides plenty of choices for ensuring that your diet contains enough fiber and protein.

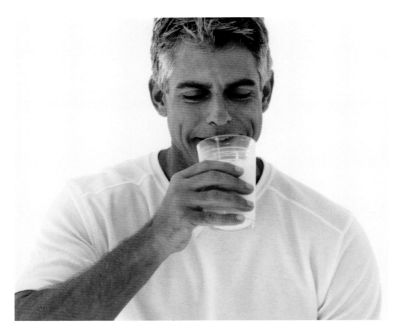

MILK
Dairy products, such as milk, cheese, butter, and yogurt, are good sources of protein.

teaspoons of sugar in tea and coffee or on cereals, cut down or do without, especially if you are trying to lose weight (see p.62).

Protein

You need protein to keep every tissue in your body, including bones, muscles, internal organs, and skin, in good working order. Some proteins are produced naturally in body cells; however, most of the protein we need to stay healthy comes from the diet and is found in a wide variety of foods, including fish, poultry, meat, eggs, and dairy products such as cheese, milk, and yogurt.

Beans (such as red kidney beans and chick peas), legumes (such as lentils and barley), and meat substitutes (such as tofu) are also good sources of protein.

All these foods contain vitamins and minerals essential to good health—for example, iron in red meat and some beans and legumes,

Beans and legumes are good sources of fiber, too. You could also try adding chick peas or green lentils to salads or making a chili con carne with extra kidney beans and cut down on the red meat.

If you are not used to eating much fiber, introduce it gradually to your diet by using both white and high-fiber foods. For example, start with a small wholewheat or whole-grain loaf and just use it for toast at breakfast (you can keep the loaf in the freezer). Try adding a high-fiber cereal, such as muesli or bran flakes, to your usual one.

Most cakes and pastries contain a lot of white flour and sugar and fat, so they are full of calories that you probably don't need. Eat them only occasionally since a lot of sugar is not good for your health. If you use more than a couple of

Q&A

Should I avoid cow's milk because it contains too much protein and drink soy milk instead?

There is no need to avoid cow's milk—if you do you will reduce your intake of calcium, which is vital for strong, healthy bones. Soy milk does not have calcium unless the manufacturer has added it. If you use soy milk, make sure to buy one that is fortified with calcium.

calcium in dairy products. Most people only need two portions of protein-rich food a day, as well as the milk in cereal, coffee, and tea. A 100g portion of roast chicken has 25g protein, 120g of salmon fillet has 15g of protein, 2 eggs have 12g of protein, 50g tofu has 11g of protein, and 230g of cooked pasta has 9g of protein.

A flare-up of arthritis, especially rheumatoid arthritis, can cause muscle weakness and weight loss. It can also make you feel generally unwell and cause you to lose your appetite, so you might need to eat smaller protein-rich meals more frequently to get the amount of protein you need.

Fats and oils

All fats and oils are high in energy and they are essential to the body's absorption of certain vitamins. They come in different forms and some are more beneficial to your health than others, so it is important to know what kind of fat you are eating.

The type known as saturated fat is found in red meat and many processed foods—for example, meat pies, sausages, hard cheese, butter, cakes, pastry, cream, coconut oil, and palm oil. This saturated fat is not regarded as a "healthy" fat because eating large amounts can increase the level of cholesterol in your blood and contribute to having a higher risk of developing heart disease.

Unsaturated fats in vegetable oils, some margarines, and oily fish are generally better for you and your heart. Today, there is so much choice it is not difficult or expensive to eat fats that may be more beneficial, particularly for people with arthritis.

Try to cut down on foods that are high in saturated fats and eat more that are rich in unsaturated fats. These include canola, sunflower, and olive oils, oily fish, avocados, and some nuts (such as almonds and pecan). (See p.56 for information on omega-3 fats, which may help ease arthritis.)

AVOCADO
Eating an avocado in a salad will help you boost your intake of unsaturated fats and cut down on saturated fats.

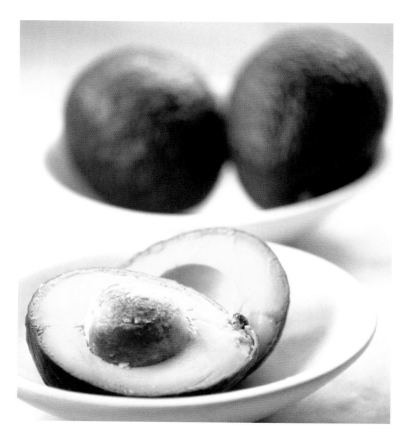

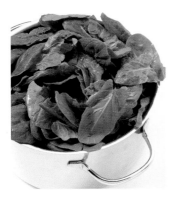

SPINACH
If you don't like to eat dairy products, spinach and other dark-green, leafy vegetables are also good sources of calcium.

Vitamins and minerals

Most of the fresh foods we eat contain naturally occurring vitamins and minerals, all of which work in different ways and do highly specialized jobs to keep the body functioning normally. We need some vitamins and minerals in only tiny amounts, while we need to take in more of others.

Most people obtain sufficient vitamins and minerals from a varied diet, but if you avoid certain foods, or groups of foods, you could be in danger of missing out on a specific vitamin or mineral. For example, if you don't eat dairy products you may not get sufficient calcium, a mineral vital for strong, healthy bones.

Fluids

Water is essential to life—60 to 70 percent of your body is made up water—so don't forget to take in plenty of fluids. You should try to drink 6 to 8 glasses (about 2 quarts) of fluid a day.

If you have difficulty drinking plain water there are healthy alternatives, such flavored water and fruit juice. You should drink tea and coffee only in moderate amounts. Some people believe that water or other fluid helps arthritis by lubricating the joints. This is not true, but too little fluid can lead to dehydration, which will make you feel generally unwell and could lead to or exacerbate attacks of gout.

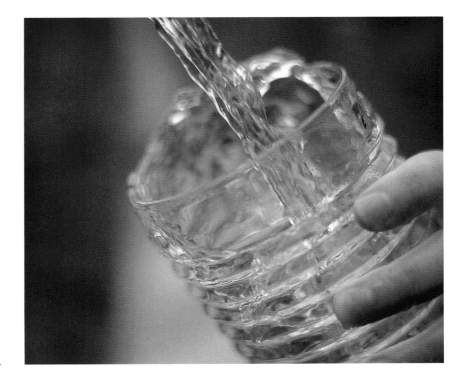

WATER
Drinking water helps to replace the water that a body loses via breathing, urine, and perspiration.

Salt

While salt is vital for maintaining the balance of water in the body, eating too much of it can be harmful—it can raise your blood pressure, for example. If you already have high blood pressure, eating excessive amounts of salt could put you at increased risk of further complications, such as heart disease or stroke.

Approximately 75 percent of the salt that we eat comes from processed food, such as prepackaged meals, soups, sauces, and even some breakfast cereals. You could easily be eating too much salt already without realizing it. (See right for information on assessing the amount of salt in a food product.)

Adults and children over the age of 11 should have no more than 6g (about a teaspoon) of salt a day. The following tips should help if you want to cut down on your intake of salt:

- Try to eat as much fresh food as you possibly can.
- Add no more than a pinch of salt to your cooking.
- Taste your food before adding more salt at the table—you probably don't need it.

Alcohol

There is nothing wrong with having the occasional alcoholic drink. But alcohol is high in calories and regular drinking can contribute to weight gain.

Excessive quantities of alcohol can, in the long term, seriously damage your health and put you at significant risk of liver disease, cardiovascular disorders, and some cancers. Alcohol is also known to provoke or exacerbate painful attacks of gout, so it is probably best to avoid alcoholic drinks if you are frequently affected by this condition.

FAT AND SALT

The information on food labels does not always make it clear whether a product contains high or low levels of fat and salt. The explanations given below will help you determine whether the food you are buying is a healthy option.

WHAT IS IT?	WHAT DOES IT MEAN?
Fat Generally, the label will say how many grams (g) of fat there are in 100g of the food. Some foods also give a separate figure for saturated fat, or "saturates."	• This is A LOT of fat: 20g fat or more per 100g 5g saturates or more per 100g • This is A LITTLE fat: 3g fat or less per 100g 1g saturates or less per 100g Between 3g and 20g per 100g of a food is a moderate amount of total fat. Between 1g and 5g is a moderate amount of saturates. Try to choose more foods that contain only a little fat (3g fat or less per 100g) and cut down on foods that contain a lot of fat (20g fat or more per 100g).
Salt Salt is often listed on food labels as sodium. A gram (g) of sodium = 2.5g of salt.	• This is A LOT of salt: 1.25g salt or more per 100g 0.5g sodium or more per 100g • This is A LITTLE salt: 0.25g salt or less per 100g 0.1g sodium or less per 100g Try to choose foods that are low in salt (0.25g salt or less per 100g).

If you do drink alcohol, try to keep to the recommended number of units per week. For men, this should be no more than 3 units a day (21 units per week) and for women, no more than 2 units a day (14 units per week). See Units of alcohol (left), which shows you how many units of alcohol are in some of our favorite drinks.

If you are a wine drinker, keep an eye on the alcohol content percentage—it can make a big difference to the number of units you drink. If you have gout, especially avoid alcoholic drinks that contain sediment, such as real ale, mature red wine, or port.

Finally, make sure you have at least two alcohol-free days a week to give your liver a break, and— above all—avoid binge drinking.

Nutrients that may help your arthritis

By eating a varied diet that includes plenty of fresh foods, you can be sure that you will get enough of every nutrient that is essential to you in good general health. However, people with arthritis may benefit from boosting their intake of certain foods and nutrients. (See also Natural Remedies and Supplements, pages 110–117, for further information on adding supplements to your diet.)

Omega-3 fatty acids

Polyunsaturated fatty acids are a group of fats that may benefit people with arthritis. One form of these—known as omega-3 fatty acids—has been found to reduce both pain and inflammation in people with rheumatoid arthritis.

The foods that contain omega-3 fatty acids are mainly oily fish such as mackerel, salmon, trout, sardines, herring, yellowtail, and eel. (White fish contains very little of the omega-3 fatty acids, although it is a good source of lean protein.)

Other sources of omega-3 are plant oils such as canola and safflower; and grapeseeds, walnuts, and pine nuts. Omega-3 fatty acids have other health benefits, too. They are good for your heart as well as your joints, and fish oil is a rich source of vitamin D, which is vital for healthy bones.

WALNUTS
If you don't like eating fish, walnuts are good alternative source of omega-3 fatty acids.

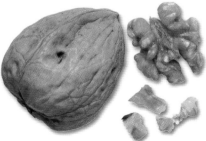

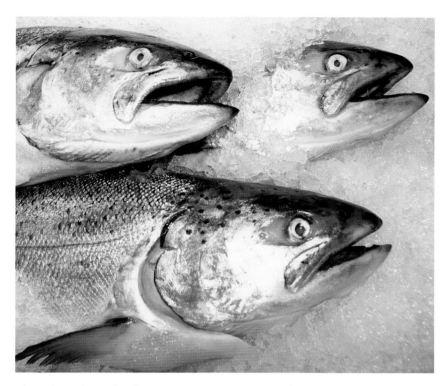

OILY FISH
Salmon and other oily fish, such as herring, trout, mackerel, and sardines, are good sources of omega-3 fatty acids.

There have been food scares in recent years about oily fish having high levels of pollutants, such as mercury, dioxins, and PCBs. Current advice from the US Department of Agriculture suggests that adults can safely eat two to four portions of oily fish a week. One portion is about 5oz (140g) of fish. However, women planning to become pregnant should limit their intake of oily fish to one portion a week. Don't eat more than one portion a week of shark, swordfish, or marlin because of the high levels of mercury they may contain (pregnant women should avoid them altogether).

Taking supplements is an easy way of increasing your intake of omega-3 fatty acids, but check the labels or ask the pharmacist for advice if you are not sure what to buy. Oils from the body of the fish contain the most omega-3 fatty acids and are likely to be the most effective supplement for people with arthritis, particularly rheumatoid arthritis.

Cod liver oil contains far less omega-3 fatty acids than fish body oils. Cod liver oils usually have high concentrations of vitamins A and D. Both these vitamins are good for you but too much may be harmful. If you take cod liver oil, limit the dose to one capsule a day and avoid taking other supplements that contain high amounts of vitamin A.

MYTH OR TRUTH?

MYTH

Some foods cause a flare-up in rheumatoid arthritis.

TRUTH

Not necessarily. Common culprits are said to be foods from the nightshade family (potato, onion, tomato, and eggplant) and various peppers and pepper-derived spices (paprika or cayenne). However, studies show that while food-related flares can occur, only a small percentage of people are affected, so such reactions are most likely to be coincidental.

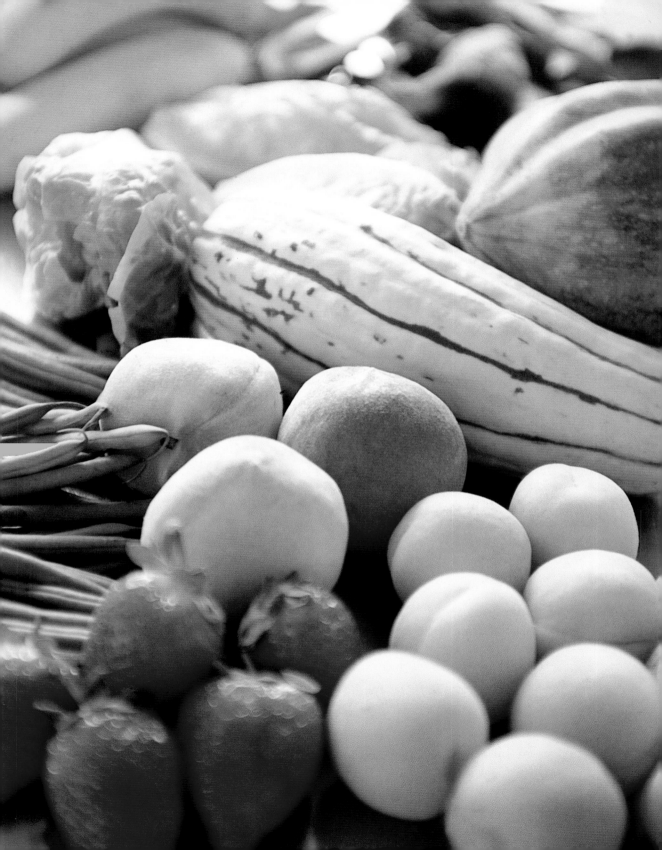

Should I avoid eating oranges and tomatoes because of the risk that the acid will cause the rheumatoid arthritis in my joints to flare up?

Many people with arthritis think that citrus fruits and tomatoes cause their joints to become inflamed. However, there really is no good evidence that avoiding these foods works for everyone with rheumatoid arthritis. What you do miss out on are tasty foods with valuable sources of vitamin C and folic acid.

Fruit, vegetables, and antioxidants

Nutrients called antioxidants can prevent or slow the deterioration of healthy tissue that results from exposure to the environment. They are essential to your diet and are especially important if you have arthritis (or want to prevent it).

Most brightly colored fruits and vegetables contain antioxidants. Good sources include oranges, kiwi fruit, corn, blueberries, cranberries, red grapes, prunes, broccoli, spinach, carrots, and tomatoes. Green tea (see p.116) is also rich in antioxidants and some research has shown that it may be particularly good for people with osteoarthritis.

FRUIT AND VEGETABLES
A regular daily intake of fresh fruit and vegetables is essential for health because of the vitamins, minerals, and antioxidants they contain.

Bananas, mushrooms, and tomatoes are good sources of potassium, a mineral that helps muscles work properly and contributes to maintaining healthy bones. Some prescription drugs used for arthritis can lower the level of potassium in the blood, so including potassium-rich foods in your diet can help counteract this effect.

Five a day

Try to eat at least five portions of fruit and vegetables a day. As a rough guide, one portion equals:
- An apple, orange, grapefruit, pear, or banana.
- Two plums or kiwi fruit.
- A slice of melon or pineapple.
- Three heaping tablespoons of mixed fruit salad.
- A heaping tablespoon dried fruit.
- 150ml of pure fruit juice.
- Eight cherry tomatoes.
- Three heaping tablespoons of vegetables, such as beans.
- A bowl of salad as a side serving.

Getting five portions might be easier than you think—just add up what you eat during the day. You could have:
- A glass of juice and a sliced banana with your cereal at breakfast (two portions);
- A side salad at lunch (one portion).
- A pear as an afternoon snack (one portion).
- A serving of vegetables with your evening meal (one portion).

MAKING THE MOST OF FRUIT AND VEGETABLES

- Eat fruit and vegetables as fresh as possible.

- Always cover and chill cut-up vegetables. Don't soak them, since vitamins and minerals can be lost.

- Don't overcook. Start with boiling water and cover the pan tightly to keep in the steam and speed up the cooking. You could also use a steamer or a microwave.

- Cook fruit and vegetables in a little water and then use the cooking water to make sauce or soup.

- Don't leave cooked fruit or vegetables food standing hot for too long because the vitamin levels start to drop within a few minutes.

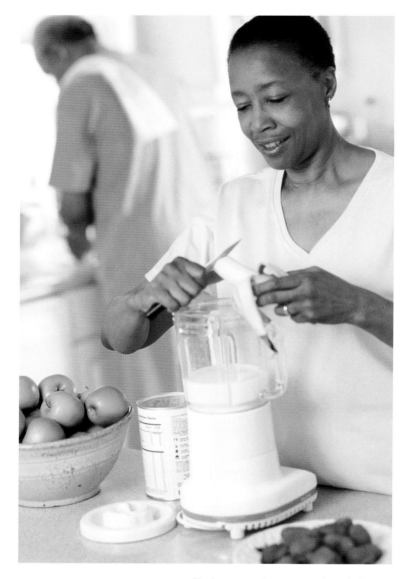

BANANA SMOOTHIE
Fruit smoothies served straight from the blender are brimming with nutrition and are an excellent way to start the day.

Good sources of calcium include dairy products (such as milk, yogurt, and cheese), certain dried fruits (such as apricots), green leafy vegetables (such as spinach and cabbage), legumes, sesame seeds, and sardines with their bones. You should try to include some of these foods in your diet on a daily basis.

Malic acid and magnesium

There is unconfirmed evidence that high doses of malic acid and magnesium supplements may bring relief from fibromyalgia for people whose muscle pain is not localized. Apples are a source of both nutrients. Magnesium may interact with your medication so check with your physician before taking high doses.

Folic acid

Folic acid, which is also known as folate, belongs to the B group of vitamins. This nutrient can help alleviate the side effects of some of the medications that are prescribed for rheumatoid arthritis, such as methotrexate and sulfasalazine (see p.82). To counteract these side effects, a high dose of folic acid supplements is usually prescribed to be taken once a week or a lower dose daily.

You can also boost your natural intake of folic acid by eating a whole range of foods. These include green leafy vegetables (such as cabbage and spinach),

Dairy products and calcium

Dietitians strongly recommend that everyone, especially women, should regularly eat foods that are rich in the mineral calcium—ideally, from childhood through to old age—to keep their bones healthy and prevent osteoporosis (see p.35) later in life.

Q&A

I have been avoiding certain foods for six months now and am not sure it's helping. How can I tell if this elimination diet works, and should I keep to it?

If you're not sure that avoiding the foods has helped, try adding them back into your diet one at a time— say once a week. Keep a diary of what you eat and make a note of any symptoms you feel. This way you may be able to tell if any of the foods are making you feel worse. If yes, then continue to avoid that food but otherwise put them all back into your diet and enjoy eating them.

beans, whole-grain bread, fortified breakfast cereals, liver, yeast extract, egg yolk, and milk and other dairy products.

Vitamin E and selenium

Vitamin E (found in wheatgerm, vegetable oils, nuts, and seeds) and the mineral selenium, found in Brazil nuts (one nut contains your daily intake of selenium), meat, and cereals, may benefit people with rheumatoid arthritis. Current research is not conclusive enough to suggest that taking these supplements is advisable. If you do take supplements, make sure they come from natural sources.

Purine-rich foods and gout

Some foods contain high levels of substances called purines, which, when broken down in the body during digestion can cause an increase in uric acid. Excess uric acid deposited in joint tissues is the cause of the severe pain felt in gout (see p.23).

Many foods are rich in purines. These include liver, kidneys, heart, and other organ meats, meat extract; venison, grouse, and duck; some oil-rich fish (such as mackerel, herring, shellfish, and anchovies); yeast (extract and tablets); and hard, extra aged cheese.

Unfortunately, many of these purine-rich foods are also highly nutritious; some, such as the oily fish, are recommended for inflammatory conditions such as rheumatoid arthritis.

If you are prone to repeated attacks of gout, particularly if your symptoms are not controlled by

High doses of malic acid and magnesium supplements may bring relief for people with fibromyalgia who have all-over muscle pain.

EGGS
The yolk of eggs contains a number of vitamins such as folic acid and vitamin B_{12} that are essential for health.

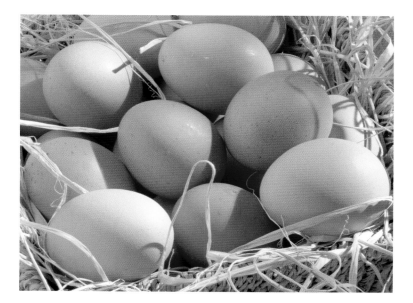

medication, then avoiding these purine-rich foods may help you keep acute attacks at bay.

Alcohol, especially beer, is also high in purines, so restrict how much you drink—or better still, cut out alcohol altogether.

Weight control

One of the most important things you can do is to keep your weight within a healthy range. Being either too fat or too thin not only affects how well you manage your arthritis but also has implications for other aspects of your health. There is no such thing as the "ideal" weight. The weight that is right for you depends on various factors, such as your height, age and level of activity.

Always speak to your physician before embarking on a program to lose or gain weight, because your medication and any other treatments may need to be adjusted accordingly. If you are a healthy weight now (see BMI, p.199), then try to keep it that way by eating sensibly and staying as active as possible.

Being overweight

If you are overweight you could be helping make your arthritis worse, since you will be putting extra stress on your joints. Excess fat is also thought to be directly linked to the process of inflammation, so

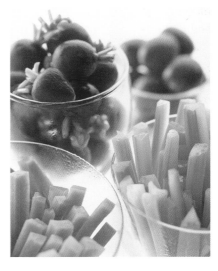

CRUDITÉS
Snack on fruit and raw vegetables such as apples, celery, radishes, and carrot sticks, instead of being tempted by the sweetness of cookies and cakes.

people with rheumatoid arthritis should be especially careful to control their weight.

Extreme overweight (obesity) is known to be a major risk factor for developing osteoarthritis, especially of the knees, hips, and hands, and it also limits the available treatments, such as joint replacement surgery. This is because people who are very overweight may be at greater risk when having a general anesthetic and also because they tend not to do as well after the operation.

In addition to affecting the symptoms of your arthritis, carrying excess weight puts an additional strain on your heart and is a major risk factor for serious disorders such as stroke, high blood pressure (hypertension), and diabetes.

Losing excess weight will help you move around more—and keeping active is important in maintaining joint health. Rapid weight loss is not advisable, especially if you have gout; a sudden and severe restriction of your calorie intake can trigger a gout attack. Fasting is especially dangerous and could leave you weak and undernourished. (For healthy eating suggestions, see Tips for losing weight, opposite.)

Being underweight

It isn't healthy to be too thin, because this can lead to problems such as weakened muscles and reduced resistance to infections. Being underweight is common in people with rheumatoid arthritis.

Unwanted weight loss sometimes occurs during a flare-up of the disease, when the metabolism of the body tends to speed up; in addition, feeling generally unwell and the effects of certain drugs can cause loss of appetite.

Elderly people with rheumatoid arthritis are particularly likely to be underweight because they have difficulty using their hands to prepare food and as a result do not get enough of the proper nutrients. (For information on devices that make preparing and cooking food easier, see p.137.)

Trying to put on weight can sometimes be harder than trying to lose it. If you are not sure what you should be eating, ask your physician or dietitian for a diet plan. (For dietary suggestions, see Tips for gaining weight, right.)

PRACTICAL TIPS

TIPS FOR GAINING WEIGHT

If you are eating to gain weight, you may risk adding unhealthy levels of fat to your diet, especially if you use whole dairy products. You should check with your physician before increasing your intake of fats and oils or following any of the suggestions given below:

● Eat several small meals during the day, rather than attempting (and failing) to eat one or two large ones.

● If you have difficulty facing solid foods, try drinking milkshakes made with fruit or eating soups with added milk or cream.

● Eat nutritious snacks between meals, such as cheese, peanut butter, and dried fruits.

● Eat fish or lean meat every day to boost your protein intake.

● Add butter or cheese sauces to vegetables.

● Don't drink too much fluid immediately before a meal—it can make you feel too full to eat properly.

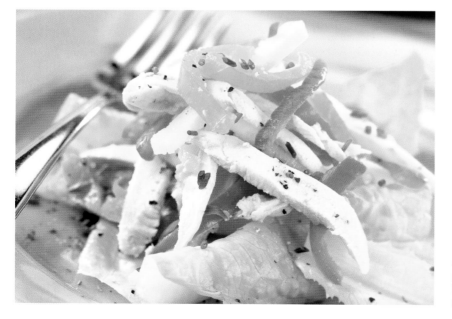

LEAN MEAT
Stir-fried chicken makes a good meal for people who need to eat lean meat every day in order to gain weight.

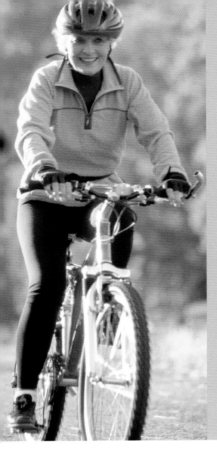

Physical activity

Exercise and physical activity are known to be very effective in reducing joint pain and disability. Yet few people with arthritis receive advice about the importance of exercising and regular physical activity.

Your joints and muscles depend on each other to maintain and improve their health and to control your movement. Regular exercise is essential for keeping your joints working efficiently. It may seem like a paradox, but simple physical activities—not rest—can not only keep your joints and muscles working properly but can also contribute to reducing your pain and disability.

Exercise and physical activity help your heart, lungs, and blood vessels become stronger and more efficient, so that you can do more with less effort.

The benefits of physical activity

Movement is good for your joints. Exercise and regular physical activity will ensure that your joints and muscles work efficiently and effectively by making them do what they were designed to do: move, contract, and work.

An increasing amount of evidence indicates that the movement involved in exercise and physical activity has many benefits for people with arthritis. The movement can reduce pain (see pp.146–151), improve muscle strength, make you feel less tired, and maintain suppleness in your joints. It can also help you restore and maintain your mobility (see 158–171).

Exercise and physical activity benefit the rest of your body, too. They strengthen bones, improve breathing and circulation, reduce stress, stimulate digestion, help you control your weight, and encourage better sleep patterns.

The perils of being inactive
Individuals who stop being active for a prolonged period of time will find that their muscles and bones grow weaker and the cartilage lining their joints becomes thinner.

Q&A

Is it true that if I don't exercise and remain inactive I will almost certainly have health problems?

Yes. In fact, people who are physically inactive are twice as likely to die as people who are active. Exercise and physical activity help your heart, lungs, and blood vessels become stronger and more efficient, so that you can do more with less effort. Other benefits include less cholesterol, better control of diabetes, protection from some forms of cancer, less depression, increased self-confidence, and greater dignity, independence, and self-esteem.

As a result, they feel tired sooner and their joints will stiffen up.

In fact, inactivity is bad for your joints. It causes both stiffness and muscle weakness, which accelerate joint damage, leading to greater pain and disability. "Rest and take things easy" may be sound advice when a joint is very inflamed and painful. However, once the pain and inflammation subside the joint stiffness, pain, muscle weakness, and disability will return and get worse—unless you resume your previous level of activity.

You may intuitively understand that movement is good for your joints—after all, it's what they are designed to do and why you have them. What may concern and confuse you is your experience that activity often causes joint pain and rest eases it. You may interpret your experience as: Pain signals joint damage caused by activity and resting prevents joint damage. Understandably, you may assume that reducing physical activity will prolong the life of your joints and make your life more bearable.

Rest, in the short term, may make you feel a bit better. But over time, you will find that everything—especially your mobility and flexibility—gets much worse.

Exercise as part of your treatment

Many people who have arthritis consider the pain in their joints to be an inevitable and incurable consequence of living and aging. Analgesics are, perhaps, the only treatment they have ever been offered. Increasingly, people with arthritis are receiving appropriate advice about the benefits of

DOING EXERCISE
Regular exercise is one of the cornerstones of health since it keeps the body in trim and encourages the mind to be alert.

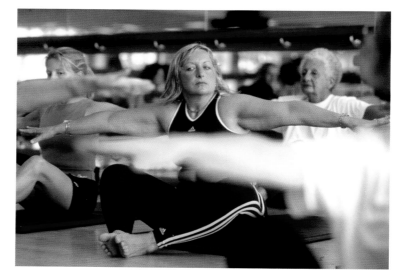

PRACTICAL TIPS

EXERCISES FOR HEALTHY MUSCLES

These exercises will help you attain and maintain an adequate range of movement in your joints and improve muscle strength, endurance, and skill:

● To regain the range of movement in a joint, move it to the end of its present range and hold it there so that you feel a slight stretch. Don't stretch it too far.

● To buiild muscle strength, do a few brief but powerful contractions of the muscle against a high resistance, such as an immovable object or a heavy weight.

● To increase muscle endurance, do many smaller contractions of the muscle against a low resistance, such as a light weight.

● To improve muscle skill, frequently practice specific activities, just as if you were learning to walk or write. The muscle activity patterns of the movement become ingrained and you can then perform them almost without thinking.

physical activity and exercise in managing their arthritis. Follow-up appointments may help reassess their condition and reinforce advice, and may even be invaluable as a means of renewing motivation (see p.72).

Relying on other treatments

Many people with arthritis do not realize the benefits of exercise and rely on other treatments, especially drugs, to help them manage their arthritis. However, some people either do not like taking drugs or experience negative side effects or have breathing, heart, circulatory, or stomach conditions that prevent them from taking drugs.

Moreover, although anti-inflammatory drugs can reduce some of the symptoms, such as inflammation and pain, they do not alter the underlying condition or prevent the problems that arthritis can cause, including joint damage, weakness, fatigue, and disability (see p.36).

Surgery can provide an effective last step but it is an option that is usually delayed—and again, many people do not want or cannot have surgery for a variety of health or personal reasons.

All in all, people have to rely on themselves to control their condition; they cannot look to their physician or rheumatologist to produce a magic cure, nor should they assume that their condition is hopeless. There is a

great deal you can do to manage your condition and become less reliant on others. Exercise and physical activity are important ingredients in this plan.

Exercise and medication

People with inflammatory arthritis, such as rheumatoid arthritis, rely on medication to help them control their disease. Continue to take your prescribed medicine and discuss your exercise needs with your doctor if you wish.

If, however, you have the more common osteoarthritis you might find you can reduce the amount of medication you need to control your symptoms. You may be able to take it when you need it to give you most relief, such as before going out, going to bed, or before exercise. Medication can make your life more comfortable and bearable and allow you to be physically active.

Used separately, drugs and exercise can help; together they can be very effective. If you start exercising you are still likely to experience times and episodes of pain, but these may not be as often, or as bad, or last as long.

Controlled exercise and even simple physical activity is good for your joints and your general health. Whatever you achieve will be hard won by your efforts, but the sense of personal satisfaction and ability to control and self-manage some of your symptoms will more than compensate.

Range of movement

Each of the joints in your body is designed to move smoothly through a range of movement (see p.12). Joints need to be exercised regularly to ensure that their range does not become restricted.

Lack of exercise will probably stop the joint from working effectively and, as a result, it may not respond fully when you need it to. For example, if you cannot bend your knees and hips fully, you will find that walking becomes difficult. If the movement of your shoulder is restricted you will find that combing your hair, washing, and dressing is more difficult. Generally speaking, as you grow older, you lose the range of movement in your joints more quickly and regain it more slowly.

Healthy muscles

For your joints to work effectively and efficiently, it is vital that your muscles are in good condition. For a joint to move, one or more of

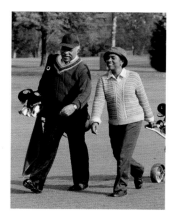

MUSCLE TONE
Playing a round of golf on a regular basis improves muscle tone and exercises a number of joints in the body.

HOW MUSCLES MOVE A JOINT

Individual skeletal muscles connect two bones together across a joint. A tendon, composed of a tough protein called collagen and wrapped in a synovial sheath, anchors the fibers of a muscle to the fabric of a bone. Each muscle has the power to contract and exert a pulling force on the bones to which it is attached. Many skeletal muscles, such as the biceps and triceps of the upper arm, are arranged in pairs on either side of a joint. The pairs of muscles work in opposition to make a joint work and move a particular part of the body. For example, the triceps muscle relaxes when the biceps muscle contracts, causing the elbow to bend and moving the lower arm and hand upward. When the triceps muscle contracts the biceps relaxes, opening the elbow and straightening the arm.

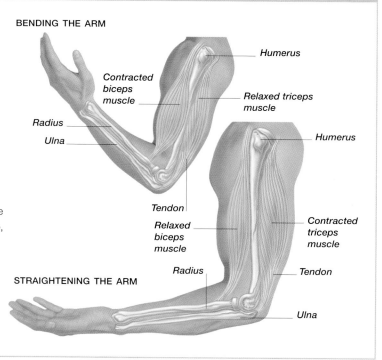

BENDING THE ARM

Humerus

Contracted biceps muscle

Relaxed triceps muscle

Radius

Ulna

Humerus

Tendon

Relaxed biceps muscle

Contracted triceps muscle

Radius

Tendon

STRAIGHTENING THE ARM

Ulna

the muscles attached to it needs to contract. Yet your muscles do not just bring about large movements, they produce smooth, finely controlled movements, too. When these two forms of muscle activity are balanced by working together they enable you to be mobile and stable at the same time.

Muscles also provide a warning system by signaling when a joint is moving beyond a safe range of movement. As a result, they can prevent harmful movement and protect against joint injury.

For example, muscles prevent the joints of your legs from jarring as you walk. The activity of the muscles around the weight-bearing joints—your trunk, hips, and knees—enables you to maintain an erect posture as you walk. Yet muscles simultaneously allow you exquisite control of the movement in these joints, enabling you to walk with a smooth gait, without jarring the joints of your legs.

Deconditioned muscles

You need to move muscles to maintain their strength and function. Unfortunately, like the range of movement in your joints, if you do not use your muscles, you lose them. Muscles that are not used regularly become "deconditioned" and unfit—they get smaller, shorter, stiffer, and weaker. Deconditioned muscles also feel heavy and tire quicker during normal activities.

The risk of joint sprains, strains, and pains increases because "unfit" muscles are slower to react and fail to signal when joints are moving out of a safe range of movement. Such muscles cannot produce smooth, finely-controlled movements, so you walk with a clumsy, uneven, and jarring gait.

Over time, this can cause pain and damage in your weight-bearing joints, further reducing their function and independence. Therefore, you need to keep your muscles in good condition in order to maintain healthy joints.

Fitting exercise into your life

With so many health benefits, why do so few people with arthritis exercise regularly? Most are never told how beneficial it can be, and the few who are told often receive advice that is unlikely to motivate them to adopt and persevere with a lifestyle change.

We all make excuses for not exercising: "I don't have time" or "It's a burdensome chore" or "It's too much hard work to get the full benefits." Perhaps you think you need expert supervision and access to expensive, sophisticated equipment and facilities.

Acquiring the full health benefits from exercise does undeniably require effort, determination, and willpower. But it does not require bouts of exhausting, strenuous exercise, nor joining a gym or using expensive equipment.

Formal and informal exercise

Fitting exercise into a busy routine can be difficult, but it does not have to be a burden. Exercise doesn't have to be "formal," such as special program in a health club. Most activities are "informal" and therefore have the same potential health benefits as formal exercise.

Walking is a very good example of a simple but effective informal exercise or physical activity that is easy to do on your own without special equipment or facilities (see next page). Even shopping, doing housework, or spending a day outdoors can be informal exercise or a physical activity.

More formal exercise activities, such as cycling, swimming, and exercise classes in a community center, are very good of course, but they require extra effort, equipment, facilities, or sometimes supervision. In reality, you can exercise wherever you like, at home alone or join an exercise class—it makes no difference.

The important thing is to find an activity that you want to do—one that is enjoyable, affordable and available. You also need to feel comfortable doing it. If you don't, you will probably soon stop. If you do feel comfortable, find the exercise level that is right for you and aim to maintain it.

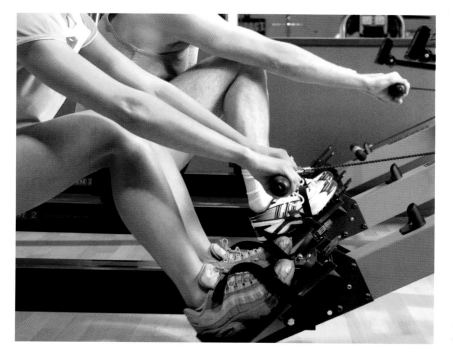

FORMAL EXERCISE
Going to the gym is one of those formal exercises that require special equipment and supervision to prevent you from damaging your joints and muscles.

Beginning to exercise

In general, people with arthritis should consult their doctor before embarking on a program of exercise. Only a very few people should not exercise at all. These are very ill people with advanced, serious, and unstable medical conditions. If you are worried or need help, ask your doctor, physical therapist, or nurse about what exercise you can do.

The vast majority of people with common stable conditions can begin exercising gently and build slowly without fear of adverse effects. Don't to be too ambitious at the start. If you are not normally active, begin with gentle exercises that are not weight-bearing—for example, slowly bend and straighten your knees as you sit on a bed, sofa, or the floor.

Over the following days, weeks, or even months, gradually increase the frequency and intensity of these exercises. Try to exercise for about 30 minutes on most days of the week. It doesn't have to be all at once—you could break it up into two 15-minute or three 10-minute periods.

Doing a little physical activity regularly is better than doing none at all. Within reason, the more you do the better. Remember, every little bit helps—you!

Your eventual aim is to practice weight-bearing exercises or activities that use your body weight as a resistance. Examples of these are stepping on and off a low step or standing up after sitting in a low

WALKING

Walking is probably the best and simplest way to encourage people with arthritis to be more mobile. However, people often find that walking increases their pain and this can be a concern.

- Make sure you are wearing good, supportive shoes or boots.
- If walking is painful, avoid long walks since they only make the pain worse. This will undermine your confidence and belief in your ability to help yourself.
- See how far you can walk before the pain starts and set a target well within this distance.
- Walk little and often within this distance at a comfortable pace.
- Rest if you need to. A walking stick may help you walk farther.

- Gradually increase the amount you walk—walk rather than drive, get off a bus earlier, take a brisk walk around the block or park.
- Each week, increase the distance a little. Vary your walks to make them interesting and enjoyable. Go with friends, alternate walks to different places, take a day off from work. and visit local attractions.
- When the weather is too bad to go out, try to do the exercises described on pages 160–71 indoors instead.
- If you do not walk regularly, start with a gentle short walk, well within your capabilities, at a speed and over distances that do not cause or increase severe pain. The next time you walk, go a little farther or a little more briskly.

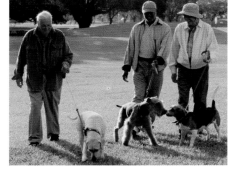

WALKING THE DOG
One way to encourage you to exercise is to walk a dog regularly. Make sure your joints can put up with the enthusiasm of a dog on a leash.

WALKING
For people with arthritis, walking is one of the best and most pleasurable ways to exercise. You don't have to stride so it is not too stressful or exhausting—simply walk regularly and comfortably.

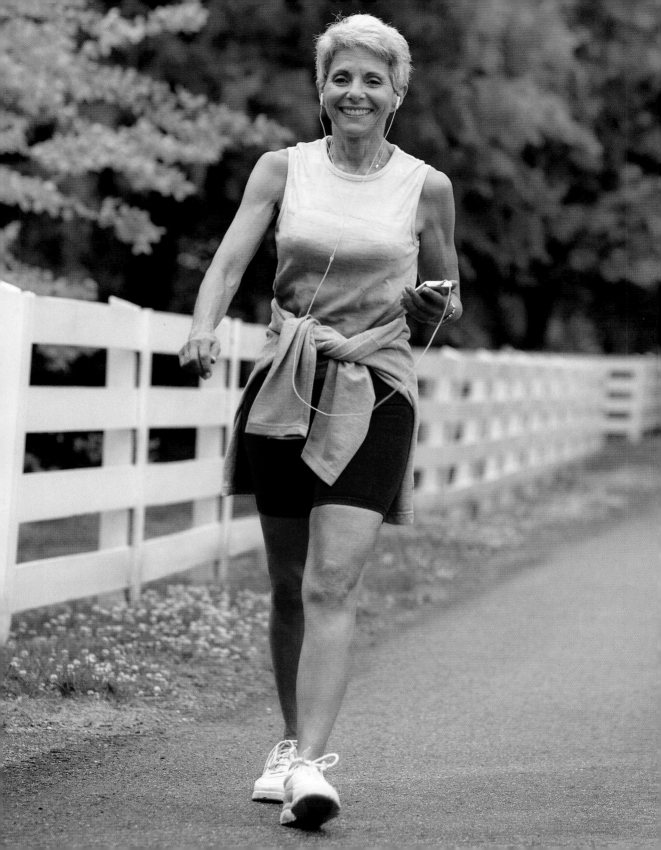

chair (see p.166 and p.169). You can also begin with low-impact activities that do not cause pain, such as a gentle walk.

Whatever exercise or activity you do, be sure to pace yourself, balancing the activity with rest, without letting the reason for resting on painful days become the excuse for being inactive on relatively pain-free days.

Stretch yourself a little

Whatever exercise you do, try to exercise near your maximum. This doesn't mean go all out and completely exhaust yourself. Rather, try to stretch yourself just that little bit more to get the best out of the exercise.

When you exercise you should feel slightly warm with your heart beating a little faster, but still able to hold a conversation—if you can't you're probably working a little too hard. How well you do an exercise is as important as how many repetitions you do.

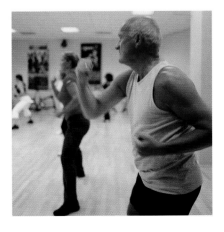

GET ACTIVE
Joining an exercise class in your community encourages you to get active and share the health benefits with others.

When you start any unusual activity, you will feel some aches or pains either during or after. If you experience increased pain or swollen joints for 2–3 days, rest for a few days until the pain subsides and then start exercising gently at a comfortable level.

Keeping going

You are likely to experience times when you cannot exercise because of pain, or because you're too busy, too tired, or the weather is bad. Accept this as inevitable but try to identify your potential barriers to exercise and plan ways to overcome them. Lack of time, pain, or bad weather may in fact be the reason you cannot exercise, but you may be tempted to use these as an excuse. Recognize this as a barrier and find ways to motivate yourself (see box, left).

If your joints are painful, then rest for a while. If the weather is bad, don't exercise for a day. But then start again. Unless the pain is very bad you can still keep going and exercise gently within your comfort zone. If the weather is bad, try to exercise indoors. The important thing is to resume exercising when the pain subsides, your enthusiasm returns, or the weather cheers up. Remember, the importance of physical activity in maintaining your health—and stay motivated.

GOAL SETTING AND ACTION PLANS

Consider your current level of activity and the impact arthritis is having on your daily life. Ask yourself what activities you would like to perform more easily if you could. You can use these as goals that exercise and physical activity can help you achieve.

● Initially, set yourself simple, challenging, but realistic goals that you can achieve within a few days or a week—and pursue them in a very focused way. They should be important to you. People with arthritis often have great difficulty performing the common activities of daily living, but being able to do them more easily can have a great impact on a person's independence, personal satisfaction, and quality of life.

● Decide exactly what you are going to do—and when, where, and how you are going to do it. Be very specific to avoid making loose plans that tend to be put off and forgotten. Write this out in a formal action plan, pin it up on the wall where you can see it every day—and stick to it. After a while exercising will become a habit.

● Tell your family, friends, and colleagues about your plan. A public "declaration" can help you carry out your "threat" to exercise. More importantly, they can remind you to do things and can become a tremendous source

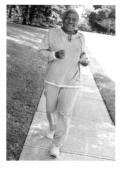

REALISTIC GOALS
Set yourself a realistic goal that is achievable, given your current level of fitness. Not everyone will be able to jog along a sidewalk.

of support, encouragement, and motivation for you.

● Monitor your progress. Circle on a calendar the days when you have exercised—and aim to cover it with circles. When you have achieved a goal, reward yourself with something you like. Appreciate how much you have improved. Tell people of your achievements—the encouragement they can give you may help keep you motivated.

● If you want, revise your goals by making those you have achieved slightly more challenging so that you are always pushing the boundaries of what you do. With a little more effort you will be amazed at how much more you can do for yourself, how much easier life becomes and how much better you will feel about yourself.

● If you can't achieve a goal, don't worry about it. Reassess the goal and aim for something less ambitious and slightly easier, so you don't become disillusioned and undermine your belief in your ability to achieve what you want to achieve.

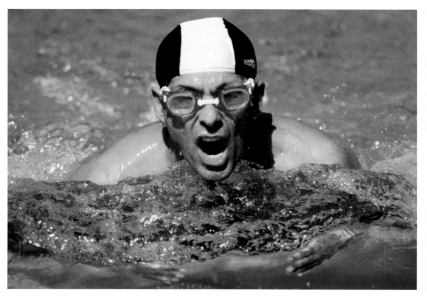

REACHING A GOAL
When you eventually reach the goal you set yourself at the beginning of your exercise plan, you will find you have achieved a level of fitness that you did not think possible.

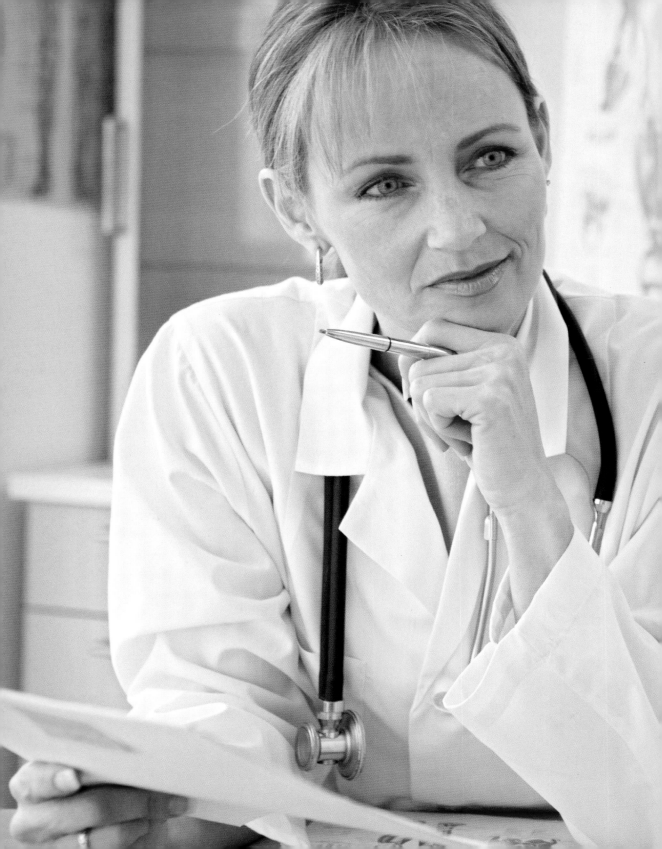

Treating arthritis

For people with arthritis the prospects for good and effective treatment are better than ever. There is no cure for many types of arthritis, but healthcare professionals can help you manage your condition so you can live life to the full.

Finding the right medication depends on the type of the arthritis you have, as well as its severity and impact on your life. Many drugs can help relieve pain, inflammation, or swelling, although deciding which is best may depend on your response to particular treatments.

Surgical treatments offer a safe, reliable option when drugs are no longer effective. Replacing joints, in particular the hip and knee, bring hope and an astonishing increase to the quality of people's lives as they rediscover the joys of pain-free movement.

Easing pain, encouraging sleep, reducing fatigue, and improving posture are among the benefits that complementary therapies may bring. If you want to try these treatments, look into them carefully with your physician. You may find that they offer valuable relief from symptoms of arthritis, especially when used with conventional treatments.

Drug treatment of arthritis

Over the last half-century pharmacologists have tried increasingly to match specific drug treatments to particular diseases. They no longer seek a magic bullet to combat all the different types of arthritis and related musculoskeletal disorders. The treatment for gout, for example, is very specific and different from the treatment for osteoarthritis, for which only less specific remedies exist. This chapter explores these treatments and highlights the potent and specific drugs available for rheumatoid arthritis.

Your doctor should be able to present both the advantages and disadvantages of drug treatment, allowing you to make your own informed decision.

Starting medication

Most people with arthritis need to start taking medication at some stage. Yet drugs are never the only treatment—rest and wearing a splint for a short time can help too, while physical therapy may strengthen muscles around an affected joint. These steps are important because you want to avoid taking drugs if you can if you have osteoarthritis because no drug is totally free of side effects.

You can buy a few of the drugs used to treat arthritis over the counter, with advice from the pharmacist who sells them. For most, however, you will need to consult your physician, who may prescribe analgesics and non-steroidal anti-inflammatory drugs (NSAIDs) in the early stages of many types of arthritis. For more potent drug therapy, your physician will usually refer you to a rheumatologist for expert advice.

In this way, your treatment proceeds in a stepwise fashion, moving from the simple drugs to the more complex, which may be given alone or in combination, according to the severity of your disease. Often, the most potent drugs will be the most expensive, so cost needs to be considered too.

Side effects of drugs

If you are faced with the prospect of drug treatment it is only natural to want to know its potential side effects. But don't forget the benefit you are likely to receive from the drug. Your physician should be able to present both the advantages and disadvantages of drug treatment, allowing you to make your own informed decision.

In this chapter, side effects will only be mentioned when they are severe. Generic rather than trade names for drugs will be used. Sometimes people fail to realize that the composition of a drug remains the same, even though it is made by several manufacturers and has different trade names.

Drug interactions

The potential for an arthritis drug to interact with a drug used for another medical condition is vast. Over fifty drugs might be used for arthritis and many thousands of drugs could theoretically be prescribed for other medical conditions.

Your physician has access to full lists of drug interactions through guides such as the Physicians' Desk Reference and will draw your attention to the most serious interactions of a drug. Physicians who prescribe drugs such as anticoagulants, which are notorious for interaction, will also provide you with whatever warnings you need.

By law, a detailed specification of a drug's interactions must be given in the package. You can also look on the internet or ask a pharmacist for advice, but do not rely wholy on either source to make a balanced decision.

Always ask your physician for advice in weighing the dangers against the benefits—you may decide that the benefits outweigh the chances of a risky interaction.

Analgesics

The simplest analgesic, available in most countries over the counter, is acetaminophen. This analgesic can usually safely be taken in a dose of 500mg up to eight times a day (normally as two pills four times a day as required) with only a slight

YOUR PHARMACIST
A pharmacist will know about the drugs you have been prescribed and may help answer your questions about taking them.

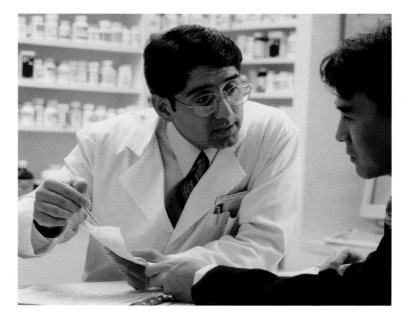

risk of major side effects. Avoid higher doses, which may cause liver damage.

Acetaminophen alone will reduce the pain of many types of arthritis. If it fails to do so and your physician confirms that you have osteoarthritis, your choice is to move to more potent pills, such as tramadol or tramadol with acetaminophen. If these fail to help, your physician could consider more potent analgesics such as propoxyphene or codeine.

NSAIDs

NSAIDs (nonsteroidal anti-inflammatory drugs) are widely prescribed because they help people with many different types of arthritis, particularly types with an inflammatory component and

where the joints are swollen, stiff, and sometimes a little hot, rather than just painful.

In the early stages of arthritis, an NSAID is usually prescribed after you have tried analgesics. NSAIDs have more side effects than analgesics, although people who need them usually find them extremely effective. Only three NSAIDs—ibuprofen, naproxen, and ketoprofen—are available over the counter, in lower doses than that normally prescribed by practitioners.

Choosing the best NSAID

Although your physician only has a choice of a few analgesics, there are many more NSAIDs that are being marketed at present. You and your physician may wish to consider three factors when you are choosing the best NSAID for you.

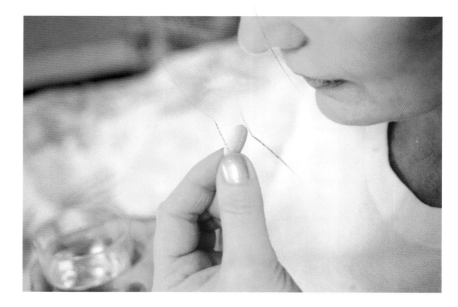

TAKING DRUGS
Drugs for arthritis are normally taken by mouth, although they can be applied to the skin or injected in some instances.

First, the family to which an NSAID belongs has some bearing on the side effects that you are likely to experience. Some side effects, notably gastrointestinal irritation, are common throughout the whole group. Most NSAIDs also probably cause a slight but reversible change in the action of the kidneys.

Second, the length of time an NSAID lasts when a single pill is taken is important. This is called the half-life. Different drugs have different half-lives—some pills need to be taken four or five times a day, others just once a day.

Third, knowing the way an NSAID works on the inflammation process that it targets can be important. Usually, an NSAID blocks the action of a particular chemical in the body, known as an inflammatory mediator.

Cost concerns

If cost is an issue, your physician is likely to start prescribing from a list of older generic NSAIDs, which are less expensive than brand name drugs.

The choice would be between short-acting drugs, such as ibuprofen and ketoprofen, that need to be taken four or more times a day; drugs, such as diclofenac and naproxen, that need to be taken two or three times a day; and drugs such as piroxicam that need to be taken once a day.

Q&A

Could I avoid the gastric side effects by taking NSAIDs as a suppository?

No, not really. Many gastric side effects result from the breakdown products of the drugs circulating in the blood rather than irritation of the stomach. Using suppositories only reduces the risk slightly and may be associated with rectal irritation.

If none of these drugs works for you and frequent dosing is found to be inconvenient, slow-release preparations of the shorter-acting drugs are also available.

COX-2 inhibitors

NSAIDs cause stomach problems because they block the action of a protective enzyme called COX-1. For this reason they are sometimes called COX-1 inhibitors. A relatively new type of NSAID, called COX-2 inhibitors, is more specific in suppressing inflammation, while at the same time it may protect the gastrointestinal tract, particularly compared to the older drugs.

Experience from several years of prescribing the COX-2 inhibitors has revealed that they could, along with the older NSAIDs, predispose people to diseases of the heart and circulation. This is quite rare, however, and many feel that if everyone on COX-2 inhibitors returned to the earlier drugs that cause gastric damage, the overall death rate from gastrointestinal effects would far exceed the death rate from the cardiovascular side effects.

It has been suggested that the risk of even a mild stroke or heart attack will only occur roughly once every 400 patient years of treatment and perhaps less frequently. Moreover, there is some evidence to suggest that there is no risk of this if these drugs are taken for less than a year.

The COX-2 inhibitors rofecoxib and valdecoxib were withdrawn in 2005; celecoxib, however, remains on the market.

You should discuss the risks of taking an NSAID with your physician. A family history of heart disease or stroke would not necessarily prevent their use, but if you have previously had one of these conditions, it may be better to take an analgesic instead of an NSAID.

Topical agents

You can buy NSAIDs (by prescription), analgesics, and homeopathic preparations as creams or ointments to apply to the skin around affected joints. These topical agents are absorbed through the skin more slowly than when they are taken by mouth. For this reason, side effects are reduced but they are not completely avoided.

There is little evidence to indicate that topical agents remain in the joint for any significant period of time before they are carried away by the circulation.

Topical applications such as Ben-Gay™ and Icy-Hot™, both of which contain methyl salicylate, may work in part through counterirritation. Capsaicin, which is the active ingredient in chili pepper skins, reduces the level of substance P, a chemical involved in transmission of pain from the nerve endings in the skin.

Counterirritants, such as methyl salicylate and capsaicin (see p.116), are administered only topically. The manufacturers of capsaicin point out that the only side effect is pain at the point of application, and people soon get used to this sensation while forgetting the pain that arises from the joint.

TOPICAL DRUGS
Some people enjoy applying cream to the affected area because they feel that they are actively doing something. Others find these creams messy and would be happy with a reduced dose of pills.

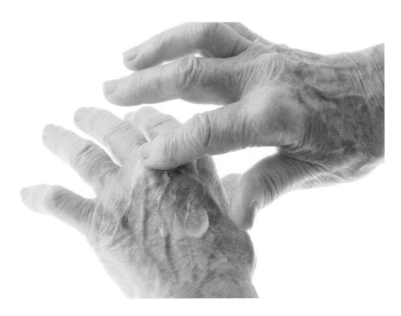

Corticosteroid therapy

The use of corticosteroids to treat arthritis is controversial among rheumatologists. Corticosteroids are very effective in suppressing inflammation but are responsible for a wide range of side effects that detracts significantly from their use. These side effects include suppression of the adrenal glands, high blood pressure, peptic ulcers, cataracts, poor healing, diabetes, and osteoporosis. Corticosteroid use makes collagen fragile, causing the skin to become fragile and easily bruised.

Corticosteroid use in early rheumatoid arthritis also remains controversial.There is a stronger rationale for using corticosteroids when the disease is accompanied by inflammation of the arteries. For some forms of arthritis, such as polymyalgia rheumatica and giant cell arteritis (see p.34), response to corticosteroids is actually considered to be one of the diagnostic criteria for the condition.

Intra-articular injections

Drugs injected directly into the affected joint—a technique called intra-articular injections—may be successful for many types of arthritis. The drug normally given is a corticosteroid, which is particularly helpful when the inflammatory arthritis occurs at a single joint. One way to reduce the risks of the side effects of the corticosteroids is for your physician to select, from the variety of corticosteroid preparations available, a corticosteroid that is relatively insoluble: it is more likely to remain in the joint for a longer period of time.

A wide variety of substances called viscosupplements, such as hyaluronic acid, have been developed for use in intra-articular injection. These substances tend to be more expensive than corticosteroids but may be more appropriate if your condition is not inflammatory. Used to alleviate the symptoms of osteoarthritis, viscosupplements may be effective for 6 to 18 months.

Treating osteoarthritis

Preventive medicine involving exercise to strengthen the muscles around an affected joint is particularly important in the early stages of osteoarthritis. Some rheumatologists have advocated using local measures, such as taping the knee cap in osteoarthritis of the knee, as a means of delaying the onset of symptoms or at least reducing them. Rest can often help, too.

Once these physical treatments have been tried, your physician will probably start you off with analgesics and then move to

Corticosteroids are very effective in suppressing inflammation but carry a wide range of side effects that detracts from their use.

NSAID TREATMENT OF OSTEOARTHRITIS

Weight-bearing joints such as the hip are particularly prone to the cartilage damage that is a feature of osteoarthritis. NSAIDs are commonly used to treat the pain and stiffness that accompanies the condition by reducing the inflammation in the joint. NSAIDs do not cure the disease, nor do they halt its progress.

Damage to the cartilage and bone tissue is followed by a response from the body's immune system and the release of chemicals called prostaglandins, which cause inflammation and pain. By stopping the production of these prostaglandins, NSAIDs are able to reduce the inflammation in the joint and reduce the pain

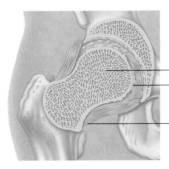

BEFORE TREATMENT
The cartilage in an osteoarthritic hip is damaged and the joint tissue is inflamed (left).

Head of thigh bone

Damaged cartilage *in the hip socket and on the head of the thigh bone.*

Inflamed soft tissue *surrounding the joint.*

AFTER TREATMENT
NSAID treatment reduces inflammation (right) and thereby helps relieve pain but only for as long as the drug is adminstered.

Pelvis

The NSAID *reaches the tissues around the joint, where it stops the production of prostaglandins.*

Head of thigh bone

Reduced inflammation *in the soft tissues surrounding the joint.*

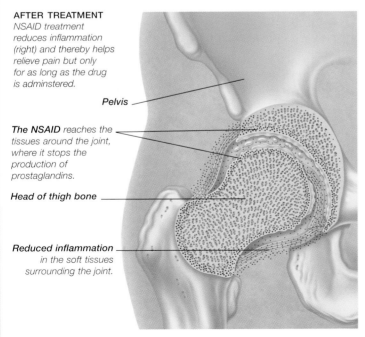

NSAIDs if analgesics alone fail to help or if there are inflammatory episodes with your particular type of osteoarthritis.

Often, the pain occurs only when you exercise, perhaps at a particular time of day, such as when you go out to do your shopping, that you can learn to predict. In this case, a drug that has a short half-life, taken just before you know you will need it, is more sensible than dosing yourself throughout the whole 24-hour-day.

Intra-articular injections and topical counterirritants often help. However, if osteoarthritis is rapidly deteriorating a single joint, you might be a candidate for surgery (which is usually successful in this condition) before the damage at one joint puts strain on others and the problem becomes more widespread.

Treating rheumatoid arthritis

More serious than osteoarthritis although less common, rheumatoid arthritis is an inflammatory condition that initially involves a joint and the tendons and tendon sheaths around the joint (see pp.18–21). As the disease progresses, however, it can involve other parts of the body, such as the eyes, heart, lungs, skin, and the blood vessels.

Many decades of research have led to the development of extremely potent and specific drugs; therefore, the management of rheumatoid arthritis has improved sigificantly over the last 10 years. There is some evidence to indicate that if your rheumatoid arthritis is treated aggressively within the first 6 months of onset, it can be better controlled.

In the very early days of your condition, analgesics are unlikely to be effective but NSAIDs may provide some relief. This may give you a false sense of security because the NSAIDs mask the symptoms but do not prevent progressive joint damage.

Such damage may be minimized by disease-modifying anti-rheumatoid drugs (DMARDs). Various DMARDs are available, including methotrexate, sulfasalazine, leflunomide, and hydroxychloroquine. They may be used alone or in combination (see p.81). If your response to DMARDs is inadequate, you may be considered for a new generation of drugs called biologic agents (see p.85). Developed since the mid-1990s, biologic agents specifically block chemical messenger that are associated with joint damage. Six are now available in the US—infliximab, etanercept, abatacept, adalimumab, anakinra, and rifuximab. More drugs of this type are likely to follow in the next decade.

One deterrent to prescribing biologic drugs is the expense. The biologic agents used to treat rheumatoid arthritis can have substantial clinical benefits but they are very expensive. The private health insurance market is now dominated by health maintenance organizations (HMOs) and other types of managed care plans aimed at containing health care costs; these health care plans may limit access to such expensive therapy.

DMARDs

The following DMARDs may be prescribed in the treatment of rheumatoid arthritis:

■ **INJECTABLE GOLD** Introduced erroneously to medicine as a possible cure for tuberculosis, gold injections were found by chance to stabilize rheumatoid arthritis. Side effects include skin rash, kidney damage, and depression of the bone marrow for which regular blood and urine checks are required. Because of this, gold shots are rarely used today in treating rheumatoid arthritis. An oral preparation (auranofin) was later developed but it is less effective and often causes diarrhea so it is also rarely used.

■ **HYDROXYCHLOROQUINE** Anti-malarial drugs were found by chance to improve rheumatoid arthritis. A very rare but important side effect of hydroxychloroquine is deterioration in peripheral and

Many decades of research have led to the development of extremely potent and specific drugs; therefore, the management of rheumatoid arthritis has improved significanty over the last 10 years.

color vision, and, for this reason, regular eye checks should be performed by an ophthalmologist. Otherwise, hydroxychloroquine is relatively safe although of only modest efficacy.

■ **AZATHIOPRINE** This prototype of a group of drugs that were developed against cancer prevents multiplication of cells. Since rheumatoid arthritis is essentially a disease in which the synovium proliferates, it was realized that low doses would be effective in the management of this condition. Side effects of this drug include skin rash, liver damage, and depression of the bone marrow, for which regular blood checks are required. The drug has largely been replaced by methotrexate (see right).

■ **D-PENICILLAMINE** Although this drug was initially developed for rare metabolic diseases, it was noted that it reduced rheumatoid factor in the blood. Trials showed that it was effective in giving partial control over rheumatoid arthritis. With the development of newer medications, d-penicillamine is not often used. Side effects are skin rash, kidney problems, and bone marrow depression, and, therefore, regular blood and urine tests are required.

■ **SULFASALAZINE** This particular medication was developed for use in rheumatoid arthritis nearly 50 years ago, when it was believed that the disease was caused by infection. However, it was only recently approved in the US for the treatment of people with rheumatoid arthritis.

Sulfasalazine is widely used around the world and, although it shares some side effects with methotrexate (such as possible damage to the bone marrow and liver, and skin rash), many feel they are not as severe. Regular blood checks are required.

■ **METHOTREXATE** Developed as a potent anticancer drug, methotrexate was found to effectively treat the skin condition psoriasis at doses that were much lower than those used in the treatment of cancer. It also improved the arthritis associated with psoriasis. Trials then found it effective in the treatment of rheumatoid arthritis.

The use of methotrexate spread from the US to Europe in the mid-1980s. Since the early 1990s, most rheumatologists have considered it the most effective treatment. The dosage is calculated according to your needs but normally averages 20mg a week. Some people prefer intramuscular injection, which can be tried if the tablets are not tolerated.

Regular blood tests are required to ensure that methotrexate does not accumulate in toxic amounts in the bone marrow and the liver. This medication may cause mouth ulcers and a rare but severe inflammation of the lungs.

■ **CYCLOSPORINE** Developed from a fungus used to prevent rejection of kidney transplants, cyclosporine was found to have some action in rheumatoid arthritis. Because it is much less effective than methotrexate or some other drugs, cyclosporine is now used less frequently. Side effects, which include raised blood pressure and impairment of kidney function, must be monitored carefully.

■ **LEFLUNOMIDE** Introduced in the mid-1990s, this drug is specifically designed for treating rheumatoid arthritis. It blocks one particular pathway in cell multiplication, thereby slowing the spread of the disease. It has proved fairly effective in certain individuals and, in many cases, it now provides a second choice after methotrexate. Side effects of leflunomide may include raised blood pressure, an increased susceptibility to infections, and, sometimes, weight loss.

Biologic agents

In the 1990s, scientists found that rheumatoid arthritis is switched on in the body by chemical messengers called cytokines, one of which is TNF–alpha. They discovered that another cytokine, known as IL–1, plays a secondary role in triggering the disease. Medical researchers have since developed a group of drugs named biologic agents to block and thereby neutralize these cytokines.

They provide a much higher degree of disease specificity than the DMARDs.

Six such biologic agents are available: infliximab, etanercept, and adalimumab block the action of TNF–alpha, anakinra blocks IL–1, abatacept inhibits T-cell function, and rifuximab selectively depletes B-cells. At present, all of these drugs have to be injected or infused into a vein.

Because cytokines play a fundamental role in regulating the body's response to disease, prescribing biologic agents has been cautious. To date, the theoretical concern that these medications would increase susceptibility to cancer (since TNF–alpha protects against cancer) has not been substantiated, although this possibility remains

Q&A

My husband and I are hoping to start a family. Will the DMARDs I'm taking affect the baby?

Yes, it is possible that the DMARDs will cause problems for your developing baby, particularly in the first trimester of pregnancy. Talk with your physician before you become pregnant and find out all you can about the risks. You may also need to discuss an alternative regime of drugs to help you cope with your symptoms until you conceive and while you are pregnant. Some people find that the symptoms of rheumatoid arthritis disappear during pregnancy.

The use of methotrexate spread from the US to Europe in the mid-1980s. For the last 15 years most rheumatologists have considered it the most effective treatment.

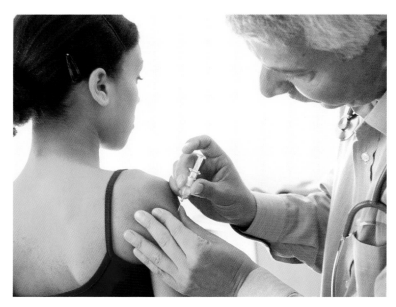

INJECTING DRUGS
Drugs may be administered by injections of different types. Nurses usually give injections under the skin or into the muscle, while doctors give injections directly into a vein, and patients self-inject.

under close review. Another concern, regarding the use of biologic agents, that infections would increase (because TNF–alpha protects against infection), has been substantiated, especially for some chronic infections, notably tuberculosis where there is a risk of awakening a previously dormant disease rather than catching the infection.

■ **INFLIXIMAB** This medication is an antibody against TNF–alpha. It is made partly in the mouse and therefore contains foreign mouse protein, which requires a low dose of methotrexate to be given simultaneously in order to prevent an allergic reaction. Infliximab has to be administered intravenously, usually at an outpatient center each time it is needed (usually every 2 months after two initial loading doses).

■ **ETANERCEPT** This competes with TNF–alpha in the body, displacing it from the places where it causes joint damage. The drug is given by subcutaneous injection, once or twice a week. It may be given with or without methotrexate.

■ **ADALIMUMAB** This is an antibody that is made independently of animals and therefore is less likely to cause allergic side effects. It is injected under the skin, usually every second week because it acts for a longer period of time than etanercept. It may also be given with or without methotrexate.

■ **ANAKINRA** This drug also needs to be given with a small dose of methotrexate. It blocks the IL–1 cytokine but it appears to be less effective. Anakinra is given as a daily self-injection.

■ **ABATACEPT** This drug is a biologic agent that interferes with T-cell function so that fewer cytokines are made. It can be given with or without a DMARD. It is given as a monthly infusion.

■ **RITUXIMAB** This drug was developed to treat a cancer called non-Hodgkin's lymphoma. It is approved for treating rheumatoid arthritis in a different dosing regimen. A course of treatment consists of two infusions given 2 weeks apart. This course can be repeated, but no sooner than 6 months later. Rituximab works by selective depletion of B-cells, which are responsible for making pro-inflammatory proteins.

Combination therapy

The expense of biologic therapy led rheumatologists to develop specific combination therapies for people with rheumatoid arthritis who had tried some or all of the available medications. One particular combination that has been found to be effective for some people involves the DMARDs sulfasalazine, methotrexate, and hydroxychloroquine.

The theory regarding this form of treatment is that remission from the disease is maintained by the combination of drugs acting on the body in different ways, and there are less potent side effects because each drug is given at a lower dose than if it had been used on its own.

When prescribing a course of combined drugs, a rheumatologist usually reviews the many separate DMARDs in turn and then proposes a specific combination on the basis of each person's idiosyncrasies. In this way, a drug that was previously discarded because it was ineffective when administered alone is tried again because it might be effective when used in combination.

The end result of combination therapy is that a proportion of people with rheumatoid arthritis who are denied biologic therapy either on the grounds of availability or because of their high cost could nevertheless receive effective treatment.

TREATING OTHER TYPES OF ARTHRITIS

Osteoarthritis and rheumatoid arthritis are the most common types of the disease. The drugs used to manage them often provide a starting point for doctors and rheumatologists who are looking to treat of other types of arthritis. For example, DMARDs are used to treat ankylosing spondylitis and lupus, and analgesics and anti-inflammatories are used for acute gout.

CONDITION	TREATMENT
Ankylosing spondylitis, psoriatic arthritis, and reactive arthritis	DMARDs (disease-modyfying antirheumatoid drugs) such as methotrexate and sulfasalazine are used for these conditions. The biologic agents etanercept and infliximab are approved for ankylosing spondylitis and psoriatic arthritis.
Lupus (systemic lupus erythematosus, or SLE)	The list of effective DMARDs for lupus is small. Hydroxychloroquine is particularly helpful and azathioprine is also used. If there is a severe accompanying vasculitis (see p.34), systemic corticosteroid therapy with or without cyclophosphamide therapy may be required. Other biologic drugs are in development to block the cytokines relevant to lupus and its relatives. A drug called mycophenolate mofetil is used to treat lupus when the disease affects the kidneys.
Gout	Analgesics and anti-inflammatory agents have a role in managing acute attacks of gout. Drugs that alter uric acid metabolism are used for long-term management of the condition. The most commonly used drug is allopurinol.
Fibromyalgia	Antidepressants taken at night, in a dose much lower than that normally needed to relieve depression, can significantly modify the symptoms of fibromyalgia during the day.

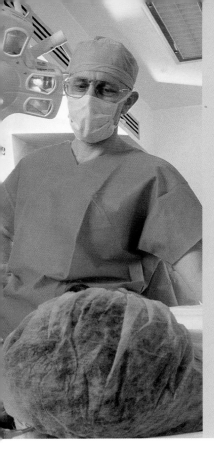

Surgical treatments

If an arthritic joint is so damaged that the pain cannot be managed with drugs or the joint can barely move, then surgery may be the only answer. Modern surgical treatments that focus on specific joints are refined, safe, and successful. In fact, joint replacement surgery—particularly of the hip—has become one of the most effective treatments in all of medicine. Surgery offers longer-lasting solutions because surgeons now place additional emphasis on preparing people prior to their operation while other health professionals (such as physical and occupational therapists) focus on improving recovery and rehabilitation.

Operating rooms are equipped with ultraclean laminar airflow systems and dedicated staff help maintain hygiene and reduce the risk of infection.

Candidates for surgery

The single most important sign that you might need surgery is the pain you continue to feel in one of your joints, despite having tried a variety of other treatments. It does not matter which type of arthritis is affecting you.

This indication means that you—and many other people who have arthritis, too—may be suitable candidates for surgery. However, while surgery is fully able to address problems relating to an individual joint, an operation will not be able to stop arthritis that affects a number of joints.

How bad does your pain have to be before surgery is needed? Two examples illustrate how the timing of surgery is crucial and why it can be a difficult decision to make.

First, a retired woman who is in constant pain from an arthritic knee, especially pain that wakes her at night, would immediately benefit from a knee replacement and its likely 15-year lifetime.

Second, an active working man of 38 with an arthritic hip that hurts at the end of a long day would get pain relief from a hip replacement. However, although the implant would allow the man to remain active, the joint would need to be replaced again (see p.107) at least once, if not more.

The person with arthritis and his or her surgeon need to discuss the risks and benefits before they can make a decision about surgery. Advice from other health professionals and the involvement of the family may be needed, too.

Who performs surgery?

Surgery for arthritis, and replacing joints in particular, is a highly specialized part of orthopedic surgery. This branch of surgery has evolved from setting fractures in plaster to treating deformities of the skeleton, replacing joints, and dealing with complex trauma.

Many orthopedic surgeons specialize solely in replacing joints, concentrating on the hip, knee, or shoulder. Training for such a speciality can take a long time—often 10 years or more after qualifying as a physician. Many large hospitals in the US and elsewhere offer specialist training in joint replacement.

Joint replacement also requires specialist facilities and expertise in the hospital. Operating rooms are equipped with ultraclean laminar airflow systems and dedicated staff help maintain hygiene and reduce the risk of infection.

Nursing staff are trained to care for the particular needs of people who are undergoing joint surgery.

Physical and occupational therapists are part of the multidisciplinary team working toward effective postoperative recovery and rehabilitation.

Surgical treatment options

Your orthopedic surgeon has a number of treatment options to choose from, depending on the particular problem that affects your arthritic joint. Replacement of a joint is one of the most common procedures; others include washing out and fusion.

JOINT SURGERY

The main types of joint surgery available to orthopedic surgeons include washing out, fusion, and synovectomy to realignment and total joint replacement. The chart below summarizes the purpose of each type.

TYPE OF SURGERY	PURPOSE
Washing out	To remove loose fragments from inside the joint.
Synovectomy	To remove the synovium from the joint.
Realignment	To correct a deformity or straighten a limb.
Fusion	To prevent joint movement.
Joint replacement	To replace all or part of a joint with an implant.
Spinal surgery	To relieve pressure on the spinal cord, to fuse adjacent vertebrae, or to remove an affected intervertebral disk.

Joint fusion is not common but it can provide excellent pain relief in the wrist, big toe joint, and ankle by preventing the movement that causes pain.

Washing out

Loose fragments formed as a result of arthritis can collect in a joint, such as a knee or elbow (see below). Often measuring at least 0.4in (1cm) in diameter, the fragments can jam inside a joint, causing intense pain and loss of movement. Washing out the joint, which has been practiced for many years—especially on the knee—can relieve the symptoms.

The straightforward washing-out procedure may involve introducing an arthroscope (a fiberoptic tube with a microchip camera) into the joint, allowing a surgeon a detailed view of the surfaces, cartilages, and ligaments. Instruments, such as forceps, remove the fragments and roughen the exposed bone on the surface of a joint (a process called chondroplasty) in order to stimulate new cartilage formation.

Some people experience relief of symptoms for a variable period of time, but there is no conclusive evidence that washing out and chondroplasty arrest or slow the arthritic process.

Synovectomy

The synovium of a joint is the source of the chemicals that cause the inflammation of rheumatoid arthritis and other types of inflammatory arthritis. Removing the synovium in a procedure called synovectomy may slow the overall arthritic process, although there is a risk of bleeding into the joint and of postoperative stiffness.

Resection of a joint

In the past, one of the few effective surgical treatments for a painful joint was to simply remove it—for example, resection of an infected hip joint, which was popularized as the Girdlestone procedure. Few joints are treated this way today, although resection of the great toe joint, especially in elderly people, may still be effectively performed.

WASHING OUT THE ELBOW

One surgical technique that may, in rare cases, be used to clean out fragments from the elbow joint is the "OK" procedure. Usually, an X-ray of the bone surfaces and cartilage of the elbow has revealed the presence of loose particles in the front of the joint. The surgeon makes a precise hole in the end of the bone in the upper arm (humerus) to provide suitable access to the front of the joint. It is important that this hole is sufficiently wide to allow the surgeon to insert instruments through the joint. Then the surgeon inserts a pair of forceps to carefully retrieve all the loose fragments of bone and cartilage.

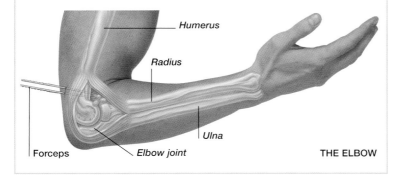

Humerus

Radius

Ulna

Forceps   Elbow joint   **THE ELBOW**

Joint realignment

Arthritis affecting certain joints of a limb may lead to a noticeable deformity. Realignment of the joint can, in some cases, reverse this deformity. The knee is the most common joint to be realigned, although the procedure can help in early disease of the hip, too.

Osteoarthritis of the knee mainly affects the inner (medial) part of the knee and is associated with a bow-legged appearance. As the arthritis progresses, more load from the weight of the body is transferred down through the inner part of the knee. Osteotomy is a procedure that can realign a bow-legged knee (see right).

The procedure can often bring about pain relief, but is only really suitable for relatively young people whose knee has a good range of movement and is not entirely affected by osteoarthritis.

Fusion of a joint

Joint fusion, or arthrodesis, may seem an odd operation for arthritis, yet it has been widely performed in the past. Two examples are hip fusion after tuberculosis-related arthritis and knee fusion after posttraumatic arthritis.

At present, joint fusion is not common but it can still provide excellent pain relief in the wrist, big toe joint, and ankle by

OSTEOTOMY

In the realignment, or osteotomy, of a knee the surgeon cuts through the shinbone (tibia) and wedges bone graft into the resulting incision. A metal plate is attached to the bone with screws to hold the incision open. The procedure straightens the leg so that the forces across the knee pass through the middle of the joint instead of the inner part. As a result, the load of the body on the knee is spread evenly across the entire joint. After surgery, the leg requires regular physical therapy to keep the knee functioning until full fitness is restored—a rehabilitation process that takes between 3 and 6 months.

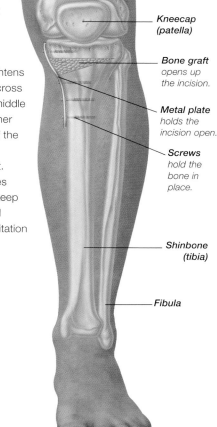

Thighbone (femur)

Kneecap (patella)

Bone graft opens up the incision.

Metal plate holds the incision open.

Screws hold the bone in place.

Shinbone (tibia)

Fibula

A REALIGNED KNEE
An osteotomy can realign the knee so that the leg remains vertical instead of leaning inward.

preventing the movement that causes pain. Problems occur because adjacent joints have to move more to compensate for the stiff, fused joint. If these adjacent joints develop arthritis early, this extra movement can make them rapidly more painful.

To achieve a satisfactory fusion, the surgeon removes the arthritic joint surfaces and fixes the bone ends firmly together until the two have healed. The techniques of arthrodesis are similar to those of fracture healing—for example, the use of internal plates and screws.

Total joint replacement

Replacing joints, or arthroplasty, is the mainstay of surgical treatment for arthritis because artificial joints can provide many years of stable and pain-free movement. The success of total joint replacement is due to improvements in surgical techniques, the methods of fixing the implants in position, and the implants themselves.

As a further result of these improvements, implants rarely break and can move with minimal friction at the surface of the artificial joint. Low friction was recognized as a key aspect of artifical joint design in the 1960s by Sir John Charnley, who is often regarded as the father of modern joint replacement.

Fixing implants

Joint replacement surgeons fix implants into position either with or without cement. Bone cement is a fast-setting polymer that binds the implant to the bone and transmits the load from the weight of the body between the two.

The polymer is applied as a viscous fluid to the bone, then pressurized to force it into the bone's porous surface. The implant is inserted and held motionless in position until the cement has set (approximately 10 minutes).

A cementless implant usually has a coating on its surface that encourages bone to grow into it to achieve a more permanent fixation. Sometimes, the use of artificial bone substitutes, such as hydroxyapatite, can enhance this process. Once a cementless joint has been implanted, bone grows into its surface over a matter of months, firmly fixing it in place.

Hip replacement

If you are in constant pain, unable to move, and entirely dependent on others, then a hip replacement can transform you into a pain-free, mobile, and independent person. Hip replacement (see p.93) has become one of the most effective treatments in medicine.

Early attempts to resurface the hip with metal molds, or to insert sheets of tissue between the rough surfaces, were not usually effective. One surgeon even tried pig bladder as a cushioning layer, with predictable results!

Hip replacement is one of the most effective uses of healthcare resources. Over 165,000 total hip replacements (THR) are performed

Hip replacement is one of the most effective uses of healthcare resources. Over 165,000 total hip replacements (THR) are performed each year in the US.

WHAT HAPPENS DURING HIP REPLACEMENT SURGERY

In a total hip replacement operation, the damaged ball-and-socket components of the hip are removed and replaced with artificial implants. The implants may be secured with or without cement (see p.92).

Removing the ball and preparing the socket

The surgeon makes a skin incision 4–10in (10–25cm) long and opens up the hip joint by carefully detaching the muscles at the top end of the thighbone (femur). Once the surgeon has separated the ball from the socket, he or she removes the diseased ball (the head of the thighbone) and the diseased cartilage lining the socket. The socket is prepared to receive either a cementless or a cemented implant. The socket is

carefully and securely positioned to ensure the joint remains stable after the operation.

Inserting the artificial joint

The surgeon inserts the artificial stem into the thighbone and fits an artificial ball to the top. The ball may be made of metal, although more modern implants have ceramic balls that are much smoother and probably wear better in the long term. The surgeon places the new ball into the prepared socket, carefully reattaches the muscles around the top end of the thighbone, and closes the skin.

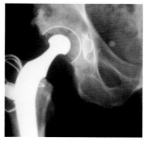

ARTIFICIAL JOINT IN PLACE
An X–ray reveals a new hip implant in position, with the stem inside the thighbone and the ball sitting in the socket.

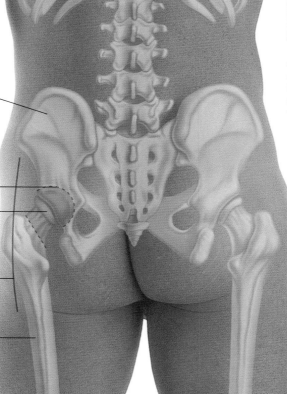

Pelvis

Pelvic socket An instrument called a reamer is used to remove damaged cartilage and bone from the hip socket.

Head of thighbone (femur) *has been replaced with an implant.*

Skin incision *is usually 10–25cm long.*

Shaft of thighbone
The center of the thighbone shaft is hollowed out using a reaming device.

PREPARING TO REPLACE THE JOINT
The surgeon first makes an incision over the hip. To prepare for the new joint, the pelvis is shaped to accept the new socket. The head of the thighbone is removed, and the center of the shaft is shaped to fit the stem of the implant.

Q&A

"After 15 years of rugged mountain biking, I have osteoarthritis in my hip. I'm in a lot of pain and even normal activities are difficult. Am I too young for a replacement?"

No. You may be a good candidate for a total hip replacement because techniques and implants have improved so much that younger, more active people are just as suitable as older, less active people.

MYTH OR TRUTH?

MYTH

Knee replacements are not as good as hip replacements.

TRUTH

This used to be the case 15 or 20 years ago when the knee replacement designs were very basic. Nowadays, knee replacements last just as long as hips, and might be doing even better!

each year in the US, and over 90 percent are successful.

In people over the age of 65, THR should have a 80 percent or better chance of lasting 20 years or more, according to the American Academy of Orthopedic Surgeons. guidance. In practice, many well-established designs of THR last much longer than this.

Resurfacing a hip joint

The technique of resurfacing a hip joint is a modern and improved version of the implants that were popular in the 1960s and 1970s.

The surgeon mills the surface of the diseased ball and fits it with a metal cap, which is supported by a thin stem in the neck of the femur. The cap fits into a metal shell that lines the hip socket. People with a resurfaced hip often regain a very good range of safe movement. Whether resurfacing techniques will outlast conventional hip replacements remains to be seen.

Shoulder replacement

The operation to replace the shoulder joint has become very important for the treatment of arthritis and sometimes for the treatment of fractures around the shoulder joint itself. A half-joint replacement (hemiarthroplasty) of the ball of the shoulder joint can produce good results.

The shoulder joint is a ball and socket joint much like the hip, although the socket is not so deep. Around the shoulder the rotator cuff muscles are very important in stabilizing the joint.

In rheumatoid arthritis, when these muscles are often in poor shape, a hemiarthroplasty is usually effective for alleviating pain. The operation may not improve the shoulder's range of movement, but the joint should feel much more comfortable.

Total shoulder replacement is usually performed when the joint is affected by osteoarthritis. The success of the procedure often depends on how much bone is available in the socket, which is usually the component that is most difficult to fix securely.

Knee replacement

The introduction of new designs of implant that more closely simulate the structure of the natural knee has revolutionized knee replacement over the past 15 years. Their predecessors were often crude designs using a simple hinge that did not allow the knee its normal range of movement. The modern total replacement is an effective treatment for arthritis of the knee (see right).

Modern knee designs perform very well in alleviating pain. It is possible that their life span may be greater than hip replacements. The risks are very similar to those for total hip replacement, so it is important that you discuss these with your surgeon before deciding to have the operation.

Replacing part of the knee

Individual parts of the knee can be replaced, too. The most common operation is the unicompartmental replacement of the inner (medial) side of the knee. Such implants, which replace only one part, can often last 10 years or more.

Less common is the replacement of the patello-femoral joint (the joint between the kneecap and the knee), although it is too early to say how successful this procedure will be in the long term.

Replacing other joints

Almost every joint in the body can be replaced, although some are more successful than others. These include replacements of the ankle, elbow, knuckles, and wrist.

KNEE REPLACEMENT

The surgeon makes an incision down the front of the knee to open the joint, move the kneecap (patella) to one side, and expose the joint surfaces. The diseased cartilage is removed, using jigs to ensure that the bony cuts are accurately positioned to receive the metal replacement the surgeon has selected. The replacement is attached to top of the shinbone (tibia)—either with or without cement—and to the bottom of the thighbone (femur), which is shaped like the natural knee to allow free and easy movement. A plastic spacer placed in between keeps friction low and allows free movement without loosening the implant. The kneecap surface may also be replaced with a plastic insert.

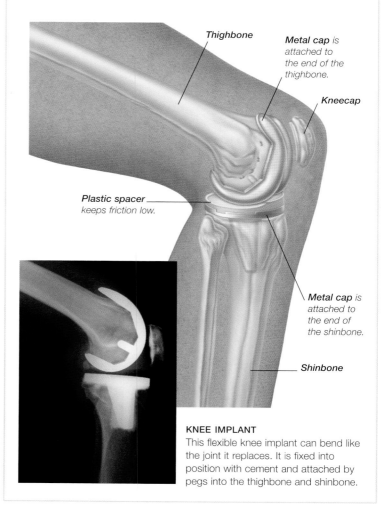

Thighbone

Metal cap is attached to the end of the thighbone.

Kneecap

Plastic spacer keeps friction low.

Metal cap is attached to the end of the shinbone.

Shinbone

KNEE IMPLANT
This flexible knee implant can bend like the joint it replaces. It is fixed into position with cement and attached by pegs into the thighbone and shinbone.

Ankle replacement

As a result of modern implants and improved surgical techniques, the replacement of the ankle joint is undergoing a renaissance, although historically it has not been particularly effective.

If rheumatoid arthritis affects your ankle, then you may benefit from this procedure. One rare risk is that, in the event of the soft tissues around the ankle breaking down and infection developing, amputation below the knee may be necessary.

Elbow replacement

As a treatment for both arthritis and nasty fractures, elbow joint replacement is improving, although only a small number of surgeons perform this procedure. If you have rheumatoid arthritis in the elbow, this surgery can bring significant improvements in your quality of life. It is rarely used for osteoarthritis of the elbow, which condition is relatively uncommon.

Wrist replacement

Replacement of the wrist joint is a very uncommon procedure and at present should be regarded as experimental. The technique may improve in the future, however.

Knuckle replacement

The replacement of one or more knuckles (metacarpophalangeal joints) is quite common in people with rheumatoid arthritis. These joints are sometimes replaced with silicone-like spacers that can give significant pain relief and improve hand function in what can be a mutilating disease.

Spinal surgery

All types of arthritis can affect the vertebrae of the spine. The spinal joints include the disk of cartilage that cushions two adjacent vertebrae as well as the facet joints at the back of the spinal column.

Decompression

When osteoarthritis restricts the space for the spinal cord or the nerves emerging from it, spinal stenosis or lateral canal stenosis will result (see p.97).

Q&A

"I have been offered minimally invasive surgery as a surgical option—what are the benefits and risks?"

Minimally invasive surgery (MIS) reduces the size of incisions as a way of limiting blood loss and muscle damage during an operation, and to improve the rate of recovery from joint replacement. There is some doubt about whether MIS for hip or knee replacement is as good as conventional methods. Risks include fractures of the femur and nerve injury. Ask your surgeon how long he or she has been using MIS and find out what the success rate is.

If the stenosis is caused by bony spurs, the surgeon can widen the space in a procedure called decompression. This involves removing tiny chips of bone to relieve the pressure on the nerves.

If the stenosis is caused by the protrusion of a disk, the surgeon may perform a diskectomy, which involves removing the protruding part of the disk.

Fusing vertebra

Sometimes considerable pain can arise from an intervertebral disk that is diseased. Fusing the two adjacent vertebrae may relieve pain, but the outcome of such surgery can be unpredictable and a failure of the fusion may lead to worse pain than was experienced before the operation.

Nevertheless, if a particular intervertebral disk has degenerated but the other vertebrae in the spinal column remain reasonably well preserved, then fusion can lead to improvements in the relief of pain.

Disk replacement

In view of the difficulties with spinal fusion, some surgeons have started developing artificial disk replacements. Some of these are based on metal and plastic, like those used in replacing a hip or knee. Disk replacement, however, is still at the experimental stage because long-term results of this surgery are not yet available.

SPINAL STENOSIS

The spine is composed of many vertebrae, each with a space in the center for the spinal cord to pass through. The spinal column is precisely stacked so that the spaces are perfectly aligned. If the space is reduced by bony spurs (osteophytes) or by the protrusion of an intervertebral disk, then pain will result. This narrowing is called spinal stenosis. Each vertebra is also designed to let the spinal nerves emerge from the cord. Narrowing of the spaces for these nerves is called lateral canal stenosis. If nerves to the legs are affected it often results in pain in the legs after walking a relative short distance, although the pain can subsequently be relieved by sitting down.

NORMAL SPINAL CANAL
The precise structure of a vertebra means that the spinal cord has enough space to sit without restriction in the spinal canal.

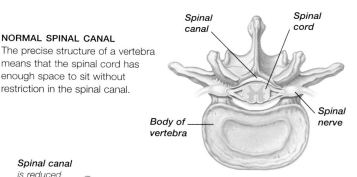

Spinal canal

Spinal cord

Body of vertebra

Spinal nerve

Spinal canal *is reduced in diameter.*

DISK PROTRUSION
When a disk of cartilage that separates two vertbrae protrudes into the spinal canal, it can press on a nerve and cause pain.

Protruding disk *narrows the space of the spinal canal.*

Bony spurs *grow into the spinal canal.*

BONY SPURS
The bone of a vertebra may grow outward and form spurs, or osteophytes. If these encroach on the space for the spinal cord or spinal nerves, they can pinch the nerves.

Body of vertebra

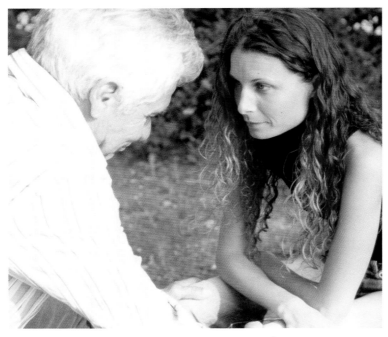

FAMILY SUPPORT
The encouragement and support of close family members can make preparing for the hospital much less daunting.

Preparing for surgery

You should consider and resolve all kinds of issues and concerns before your surgery so that you are fully prepared for everything that surgery entails. This involves resolving medical problems so that you are fit for surgery, anticipating and organizing your work and care needs after surgery, making sure that your finances are in order, and attending a preoperative assessment clinic (see p.100).

Resolving medical problems

Most surgical procedures for arthritis are planned in advance (it is often called "elective surgery"), so you have more than enough time to prepare thoroughly. Surgical success relies in no small part on careful preoperative preparation, which identifies and treats potential problems, such as high blood pressure, diabetes, and asthma before the surgery.

Efforts to reduce weight will improve general health, enhance the prospects of recovery from surgery, and may increase the lifespan of an artificial joint. The surgical process itself is also easier if you are not overweight.

Preparing for life after surgery

Before you undergo surgery, it is wise to consider what life will be like after you have recovered. Discuss with your surgeon the kind of restrictions you will need to impose on your work and lifestyle activities.

Find out what benefits you are entitled to (see p.135) and ask an occupational therapist what aids you may need. Talk to your employers before you plan any time off for surgery, so that they know well in advance about your potential absence—you can also find out about your eligibility for sick pay.

■ **OFFICE JOB** You may be able to return to work 6–8 weeks after surgery if your job does not put too much pressure on your joints. Depending on your profession and responsibilities, you may also be able to work from home. Full function may not be achieved for 12 weeks.

■ **HEAVY MANUAL WORK** If your job involves heavy lifting and carrying, talk to your employer about making modifications (see p.135) to reduce the stress on your new joint. The heavy work involved in occupations such as building or farming place especially large loads on artificial joints and will reduce their lifespan as a result. You may even need to seek alternative employment.

Arranging for care

Everybody who has surgery for arthritis will need some sort of help after the operation. Discuss your postoperative care in detail at the preoperative assessment clinic (see p.100) so that appropriate arrangements can be made.

For example, if you have a simple arthroscopic washout (see p.90), you will probably require help around the home for the first 24–48 hours, then you will need to take about a week off from work. Young fit people who have more extensive surgery will also require help for longer, at least until they recover from the fatigue they will inevitably feel.

Elderly people will require much more care after joint replacement surgery. Climbing stairs and steps as well as bathing and dressing may be difficult in the first few weeks. Family and friends may be able to help out, but home nursing may also be necessary if no family help is available. In some circumstances a short period of convalescence in a suitable nursing home may be necessary after discharge from the hospital.

Financial arrangements

Depending on what type of health and hospitalization insurance you have and who your surgeon is, most of the expenses may be billed directly to your health insurer, and you will be billed only for the "deductible" costs not covered by insurance. Alternatively, if your surgeon does not participate in your health plan or does not accept payment from the insurance company, you may need to pay for most or all of the expenses, but you can then submit them to your insurer for reimbursement.

Some insurance plans require preapproval of costs before any major surgery; make sure that you submit the appropriate paperwork before your surgery.

Finally, any medical costs that are not covered by your health insurance may be deducted from your federal income tax if the expenses add up to a certain percentage of your income, so keep careful records of all the bills.

Other expenses: you may wish to arrange for paid help to look after your house and to take care of your pets. You may also want this help to continue after you have been discharged until you are fully recovered.

PRACTICAL TIPS

GETTING FIT FOR SURGERY

● Get as much exercise as you can to improve your fitness and strengthen the muscles around your joints.

● If you have breathing problems, such as asthma, try to make sure your chest is as good as it can be. If you're a smoker, stop.

● If you are overweight, try to shed some extra pounds.

● Try to avoid infections. This includes dealing with bad or loose teeth and infected toenails.

● If you are a woman on oral contraceptives, you may wish to stop taking them because they increase the risk of a blood clot. Consult your surgeon.

The preoperative assessment clinic

The preoperative assessment clinic is a vital part of the preparation for your surgery. Be prepared to stay for 3–4 hours. You will meet your surgeon and the preoperative assessment team, which includes physical therapists, nurses, and occupational therapists.

The assessment can detect risk factors, such as high blood pressure, heart disease, and diabetes. By treating problems before surgery the team will reduce the risk of complications such as heart attacks, chest infections, and urinary infections.

■ **TESTS AND CHECKS** The team will take your detailed medical history, conduct routine blood tests, and may record an electrocardiograph (ECG) to check your heart. They may also take X–rays of your troublesome joint.

■ **INFECTIONS** Since infection is such a serious complication of joint replacement surgery, you should make sure that you are clear of any infections.

■ **REHABILITATION** Physical and occupational therapists will talk to you about detailed aspects of your rehabilitation.

The occupational therapist will be particularly concerned that any modifications to your home are done before you are discharged from the hospital. For example, you may need handrails fitted beside your bath or shower, or extra banisters installed on the stairs. If you are having a hip or knee replaced, your seats and chairs at home will need to be measured so that, if necessary, they can be raised before you return. A toilet seat may also be raised so that you don't have to bend the new joint too much in the first few weeks after discharge.

■ **BONE BANK** If you are having your hip replaced, you can donate the ball of your hip to a bone bank. It will be deep-frozen and treated to eliminate infection so that it can be used as a bone graft for people undergoing complicated revision surgery (see p.107), where they may have lost bone as a result of joints becoming loose.

If you agree to donate your bone, your blood will be tested for infections, such as HIV, but you will be counseled thoroughly about the implications of this.

Admission

When you are admitted to the hospital for surgery, the admissions staff will take you to the appropriate ward and one of the nurses will check that all your preadmission details are correct. Depending upon the time of your admission, and the proposed time of your surgery, you should not have anything to eat or drink for six hours before the operation.

It is very common for hip and knee operations to be performed under a spinal anesthetic so that you are numb from the waist down.

The consent form

Once you are comfortable, a member of the surgical team will visit you and mark the joint that needs surgery, as a fail-safe mechanism to avoid mistakes. The consent form, which you may have signed at the preoperative assessment clinic, will be checked.

This form is very important because it records the discussion that you had with your surgeon, and confirms that you are happy to undergo the procedure and understand the risks involved.

Anesthetic techniques

Modern anesthetic techniques allow joint surgery to be very comfortable, with very little postoperative sickness or nausea. You will have an opportunity to discuss with your anesthetist exactly what technique is best for you, depending upon whether you want to be awake or not during the procedure, and taking into account any other medical factors or previous anesthetic problems.

A traditional general anesthetic (GA) is still often used for joint replacement surgery, but it may be supplemented by local anesthetic nerve blocks to numb the site of the operation.

Spinal anesthetic

It is very common for hip and knee operations to be performed under a spinal anesthetic so that you are numb from the waist down. This technique has the advantage of giving very effective postoperative pain relief, and you can choose either to be completely awake during the operation or to have some sedation to allow you

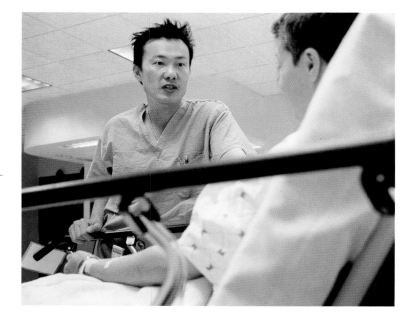

PREOPERATIVE TALK
Before you are due to go into the operating room, your surgeon will visit you. If there is anything more you need to know, now is the time to ask.

You should come around after the operation with little or no pain, and the recovery staff are there to ensure that your recovery is smooth and pain-free.

to sleep. Many patients prefer the latter, since they do not like to listen to the noise of the operating room. Much upper limb surgery can also be done under local anesthetic nerve blocks, with or without sedation or a general anesthetic. A spinal anesthetic can make urinating after the operation difficult so you may need to have a catheter inserted into your bladder.

Avoiding blood transfusions

Surgeons and anesthetists are constantly looking for ways to improve the safety of elective surgery. One particular topical area at the moment is the avoidance of blood transfusions. A blood transfusion carries a very small risk of infection and can suppress the body's natural defense mechanisms. In other words, a

---

Q&A

"I would like to stay awake during my operation so that I can watch— is this a good idea and what sort of anesthetic will I need?"

Talk to your surgeon as well as other people who have watched their own operation before you make up your mind. Watching may make you feel nauseous and increase your anxiety. On the other hand, it may comfort you to feel a part of what is going on. You will be given a local anesthetic so that only the area around the site of the operation becomes numb.

---

blood transfusion might increase the chance of a postoperative infection. A healthy blood count at the preoperative assessment will reduce the need for a postoperative blood transfusion.

Saving blood lost at the time of the operation and returning it afterward, particularly in knee replacements, may also reduce the need for a blood transfusion.

The day of surgery

When the time comes for your surgery, you will put on a gown and remove jewelry (except wedding rings), nail polish, and dentures. You may have a premedication to relax you. You will go to the operating room reception either in a wheelchair or on a cart. You go to the anesthetic room outside the operating room where you will see your anesthetist again and your surgeon will check you over just prior to the operation starting.

Coming around after surgery

When the operation is over you will return to the recovery ward either on your hospital bed or on a cart. You will have an intravenous drip in one of your arms, and you may have drain tubes connected to drain bottles, which collect any blood lost after the operation. You should come

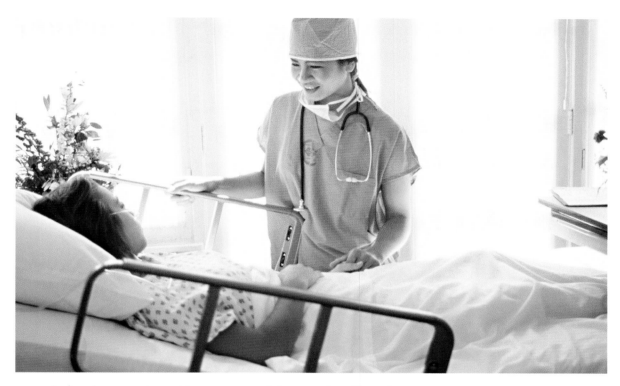

around after the operation with little or no pain, and the recovery staff are there to ensure that your recovery is smooth and pain-free. You will probably return to your room within an hour or two of entering recovery, and later in the day you should be able to have short visits by friends or relatives.

Recovery

IV drips and drains are usually removed within the first 24 hours after surgery, and you will be helped out of bed by the nursing staff or physical therapists at this stage. If you have had an operation on your arm, physical therapy can

start right away, but if you have had surgery on your legs you will be gently mobilized with the physical therapists to start with.

Recovery milestones

If you have had lower limb surgery the milestones you need to achieve in the hospital include walking safely with crutches or a walker, getting into and out of bed, and getting into and out of a chair. The physical therapists will check if you can negotiate stairs and steps.

Once you have passed all these milestones it will be safe for you to go home. Some outpatient physical therapy, especially after knee replacement, may be needed. If you have had a knee operation,

WAKING UP
After your operation you will probably feel tired and weak, but be reassured that nurses are always present to monitor and help with your recovery.

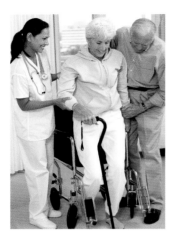

GETTING BACK ON YOUR FEET
Physical therapists will need to
know that you have reached all
the recovery milestones before it
is safe for you to go home.

the physical therapists will want to
see the muscles around the knee
recovering and to know that you
have regained a good range of
movement prior to your discharge.

At the time of discharge

Discharge planning is important to
make sure the outcome of your
operation is as good as possible.
Dissolving stitches are often used,
but if you have stitches (sutures)
that need removing, arrangements
will be made for their removal by
your physician or a nurse.

At the time of discharge, checks
will made to ensure that all the
necessary modifications to your
home are in place, and that any
home nursing care is ready for
you when you get home. The
hospital should also give you
contact numbers to call if you
do have any problems after
your discharge.

Rehabilitation milestones

When you get home from the
hospital you will probably feel
very tired, no matter what surgery
you have had. Rehabilitation
milestones will vary, however. For
example, an arthroscopy on your
knee will probably make walking
uncomfortable for the first few
days, but you should be able to
return to work after perhaps a
week or 10 days.

Milestones for total hip or knee replacements

A total hip replacement or total
knee replacement will probably
mean that you have to keep using
your crutches for perhaps 4–6
weeks after the operation. This
period may seem like a long time
but it will give both your muscles
and your wound a chance to heal.
You will then start coming off
crutches gradually, perhaps onto a
cane, but you should notice that
your level of mobility is improving
steadily.

Discuss with your surgeon when
you can start driving your car
again. It is usual to wait 4–6
weeks after lower limb joint
replacement surgery.

As long as you do not have
many other joint problems, you
will be probably off canes and
crutches completely by 10–12
weeks after the operation. At this
stage you should be walking freely
and starting to get back to a
normal life.

It is important during the
recovery from lower limb joint
replacement to walk a little each
day, to help your recovery and
minimize swelling in your leg.
You will be able to take short car
trips as a passenger almost
immediately after discharge from
the hospital, but if any longer
trips are planned within the first
12 weeks after surgery, you should
stop regularly to get out and
stretch your legs.

Complications during rehabilitation

A few complications can develop after any surgery and during rehabilitation, but the risks that are particular to the surgery of arthritis include infection, blood clots, and dislocation. There are a couple of rare complications, too.

Long-term monitoring and follow-up is important to the early identification of problems that may develop with a replaced joint (see Revision surgery, p.107).

Infection

In orthopedic surgery, infection in an implant or bone can be very difficult to treat without further surgery. However, the risk of infection is not high—in total joint replacements, for example, it is about 1 in 200.

Every effort is made to reduce the risk of infection during elective orthopedic surgery. You receive antibiotics and your operation is performed in a special ultraclean operating room by a team wearing special surgical suits.

After your operation, bacterial infections that form pus must be treated promptly to stop the germs from spreading in your blood and attaching to the joint replacement.

However, if bacteria do enter a joint replacement, they can stick to the implant. Since antibiotics have no effect at this stage, the only way to eradicate the bacteria is to remove the infected implant, let the infection clear, then insert another new implant. This two-stage approach often requires 8–12 weeks between the two stages, and is obviously a major undertaking.

Discuss with your surgeon and dentist whether you should have a single dose of antibiotics before having significant dental work.

Blood clots

The risk of a blood clot (deep vein thrombosis, or DVT) developing in one of your legs is about 1 in 20, especially after an operation on your legs or pelvis. Reducing your weight before surgery, and getting mobile soon after surgery, can lower the risk. A blood-thinning agent such as heparin can help prevent blood clots, too. You may also be encouraged to wear special support stockings or intermittently inflating boots to prevent blood from pooling in your legs.

Q&A

"How soon will I be able to fly?"

It is probably not a good idea to fly until 12 weeks after your surgery because of the slightly increased risks of blood clots (deep vein thrombosis). Many people notice that their joints continue to improve for at least 12 months after the operation, at which stage they almost forget that they have ever had the operation.

Q&A

"If I take a blood-thinning agent such as warfarin, what happens if I cut myself?"

You should contact your physician at once if you cut yourself or have a nosebleed or notice blood in your urine. Your physician will probably prescribe a drug that helps your blood clot.

Blood clots can be treated and usually do not lead to long-term problems. In some circumstances, however, the blood clot can reach the lungs (a pulmonary embolism) and may be life-threatening.

Dislocation

If you have had a total hip replacement, there is a small risk that your new joint may dislocate, where the ball and socket of the new joint come apart. This risk, which is probably only 1 or 2 in 100, is highest in the first 6–12 weeks after your operation.

It is important to follow the advice of your physical therapists and avoid getting your limb into a situation where dislocation may occur. Of course you can use the joint, but respect it and avoid overloading it repeatedly or forcing it into awkward positions. If you have had a total hip replacement, don't cross your legs or bend too far too soon. If you have had a knee replacement, don't kneel on it.

The younger you are when you have your hip or knee replaced, the shorter time it is likely to last, since younger people use their joints more vigorously.

Rare complications

If you have surgery on a limb there is an extremely low risk of a nerve injury. Your surgeon will probably explain this to you during the preassessment (see p.100).

Another rare complication is excessive bleeding after your joint replacement operation. This can result from an injury to a major blood vessel.

Long-term outcome

All replacement joints should last for many years, especially if you look after it. Studies of large numbers of people with joint replacements give statistical chances of how long a joint will last. For example, data from the US suggests that many hip replacement have a better than 80 percent chance of lasting 20 years or more, before they need to be replaced (see below).

The younger you are when you have your hip or knee replaced, the shorter time it is likely to last, since younger people use their joints more vigorously.

Knee replacement is now as good as hip replacement, and similar survivorship figures are reported. Upper limb joint replacements are obviously not under as much load as lower limb joints, and, therefore, shoulder and elbow joints may last for many decades.

Revision surgery

If your new joint begins to fail, it is usually because the joint loosens inside the bone. The load-bearing surface of the implant also wears slowly. This is to be expected since a hip or knee may go through a million movements each year in normal use. As a result, you may be a candidate for repeat surgery and a new joint.

An X-ray will enable your surgeon to detect what is wrong with the artificial joint. As it loosens, it might become painful. Sometimes, a joint can loosen without pain so that you are unaware that the bone around your implant is becoming very thin. For this reason, your joint replacement should be X–rayed every 5 years or so, even if you feel absolutely fine.

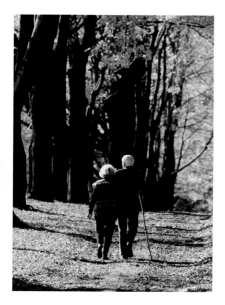

If your replaced joint loosens, you may need a revision. Surgical revision techniques have developed considerably in the last 20 years. It is possible to rebuild worn-out joints with new ones, using bone grafts to fill areas where the bone has become very thin or weak. A joint can be revised several times in theory, depending on how much bone is left after the old joint is removed and how much scarring of the soft tissue has occurred.

Risks of revision

Revision surgery takes longer, is technically demanding, and is usually performed by specialists. Nevertheless, a successfully revised joint can perform almost as well as the first one, giving you back your mobility and independence.

The risks of revision surgery are higher than those for the primary operations. Candidates for revision are older than when they had their first operation and their general health may not be as good.

For each subsequent revision operation, the risks of infection go up. The muscles, ligaments, and skin become more scarred and fail to heal as well. Blood loss can be greater and surgeons rely more on saving blood cells (see p.102).

A BRIGHT FUTURE
Total joint replacements should last for a long time without causing any problems, allowing you to enjoy a bright future with plenty of activity.

Complementary therapy options

In addition to exploring conventional treatments for your arthritis, you may decide to investigate some of the complementary therapies available now. Used wisely, these may help relieve certain symptoms, or simply contribute to your sense of well-being. You will find a great variety within the therapies. Some, such as herbal medicine, have been around for a long time, while others are relatively new. But the "complementary" part is key: the therapies complement, rather than replace, your regular treatment.

Since the mid-1990s, the market for complementary therapies has expanded at an unprecedented rate.

Therapies that treat the body and mind

Complementary therapies usually focus on treating the body and mind—in other words, the whole person. Practitioners of these therapies do not impose treatment but instead encourage healing to come from within the individual, who is an active participant. This holistic approach is based on the idea that health comes from a balance between the mind, body, and surrounding world. Any "imbalances" between these can result in poor health, low energy, or specific illnesses.

How therapies help

Pain is perhaps the primary symptom of arthritis and one of the most complex areas of human biology. We still do not know why some people experience more or less pain than others, although most physicians agree that state of mind can have an effect.

Some complementary therapies may simply help you relax, reduce stress, or encourage sleep, which in turn may help relieve pain. Side effects are a common problem with some conventional drugs and this may prompt people to explore other ways of managing their disease.

The rise in popularity of the therapies

Since the mid-1990s, the market for complementary therapies has expanded at an unprecedented rate. Walk down almost any street and you will see the evidence of this, whether it is practitioners offering their services or the enormous range of herbs and supplements that are available from supermarkets, health shops, pharmacies, and other stores.

But unlike the tightly controlled world of conventional medicine, it is a market that is largely without regulation and safeguards for the public are not automatically in place. While physicians, for example, spend a number of years studying and gaining practical, supervised experience, practitioners of some complementary therapies do not necessarily do so and may freely start a business without any medical background or training.

A lack of hard evidence about the safety and effectiveness of many therapies has led some of the established medical profession to remain sceptical about their validity. The good news is that universities and government agencies are spending an increasing amount of time and money on research into particular therapies, which should help establish better evidence-based practices in the future. Such developments may help bring better safeguards into the practice of complementary therapies.

Controls on the sale of supplements

In an attempt to regulate the more unscrupulous parts of the health market, many countries are starting to control the sale and quality of herbs and supplements. The 1994 Dietary Supplement Health and Education Act (DSHEA) stipulated the formation of an independent dietary supplement commission to report on the use of claims in dietary supplement labeling, as well as setting new standards for labeling. When checking the labeling, look for ingredients in products with the U.S.P. designation, which indicates that the manufacturer followed standards established by the U.S. Pharmacopoeia.

Categories of therapy

Broadly speaking, the hundreds of different complementary therapies can be grouped into three categories: natural remedies and supplements, bodywork therapies, and movement therapies.

However, this does not mean you can try only one therapy at a time. You can mix and match; for example, you can take a supplement and try a bodywork therapy or movement therapy.

MYTH OR TRUTH?

MYTH

If something is natural, it must be safe.

TRUTH

There are many dangerous substances within nature and, just as with any conventional medicine, you must always follow the recommended dosage of a natural remedy.

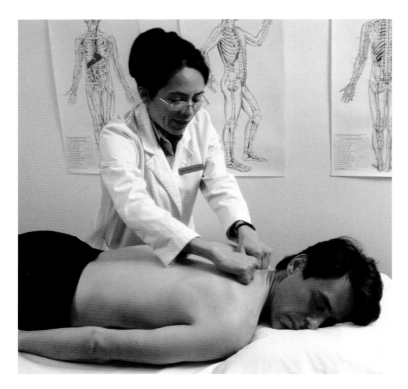

BODY MASSAGE
A professional massage can work wonders for easing aches and pains, relieving stress, and improving your overall feeling of health and well-being.

■ **NATURAL REMEDIES AND SUPPLEMENTS** Usually produced from substances found in nature, natural remedies and supplements are not yet as strictly controlled as conventional medicines. As a result, there may be a big difference between their quality, effectiveness, and safety.

Since certain supplements and herbs can sometimes interfere with the actions of drugs you may be taking, and because not all natural remedies are suitable for everyone, it is vital to choose reliable brands and to speak to your physician before you try anything. See pages 112–119 for more information.

■ **BODYWORK THERAPIES** This group encompasses those therapies that are sometimes referred to as "touch therapies," where a practitioner uses a hands-on approach to treatment. All involve work with one or more parts of the body, whether through manipulation (such as massage), touching techniques (such as reflexology), or use of implements (such as acupuncture). See pages 120–125 for more information.

■ **MOVEMENT THERAPIES** This group of therapies is based on learning to use your body to promote strength and wellness. Practitioners will teach you how to carry out the relevant exercises or movements. Usually, the therapies are not just systems of exercise but also use the mind to help facilitate body harmony. See pages 126–131 for more information.

Finding a reputable practitioner

The qualifications required of complementary practitioners varies according to the specialty. Practitioners wishing to be listed with a professional body must adhere to certain standards, such as completing a certified level of training. Many of the more established complementary therapies have some degree of self-regulation, administered by their own professional bodies. For a list of certified practioners and the certification requirements, go to the web site for that speciality, such as the National Certification Commission for Acupuncture and Oriental Medicine (www.nccaom. org). Furthermore, licensing requirements for practitioners of alternative therapies varies by state; some states have more restrictions, while others, such as Minnesota and California, allow any certified practioner to practice without being licensed.

Asking your physician about complementary therapies

Although some physicians remain very sceptical about the validity of complementary therapies and their place in the delivery of health care, an increasing number of

Q&A

How much do complementary therapies cost?

The prices that you may expect to pay vary enormously, depending on the therapy, the practitioner, and where you live. The cost of a therapy may also depend on whether you have a course of treatment or a single session. Your first appointment is often the longest and most expensive session. Always ask at the beginning what the treatment will cost, whether any supplements or remedies will be included in the price, and how many treatment sessions you may need. Some alternative therapies are covered by certain health insurance plans.

physicians recognize their value in the treatment of arthritis and the pain associated with the condition. Movement therapy and acupuncture seem to be the most effective types of complementary therapies for people with arthritis.

If you have heard that a specific therapy may be able to help your arthritis, the best first step is to talk to your physician, who may be able to recommend an experienced practitioner in your locality. In fact, your physician may even be the first to suggest a therapist as part of your treatment.

In addition, some physicians are themselves trained in a particular therapy, such as manipulation or acupuncture. It is also common for hospital pain clinics (see p.47) to offer complementary health services to patients.

Keeping your physician informed

If you are trying a complementary therapy, make sure you keep your physician or rheumatologist informed. They can tell you if a particular herb or supplement is safe to take at the same time as any existing medication; they will also know whether a therapy will suit your level of overall health and mobility. It may help to take notes of any changes a therapy brings to your health, whether good or bad, which you can then discuss with your physician.

PRACTICAL TIPS

LOOKING ONLINE

Many people turn to the internet and look online for information about health. Much of it is accurate, and useful, but some websites are unreliable. There is little or no regulation about health information on the internet. But there are ways you can stay safe:

● Check the credentials of the organization concerned. These should be clearly displayed on the website.

● Check whether the website meets the requirements of the Health on the Net (HON) code of conduct; if it has been, it can display the "HON" logo at the bottom of its home page.

● Be wary of advice that seems to contradict information you have been given by your physician.

● Be cautious of websites that are selling products or services. It is harder for such sites to be impartial.

● Go to www.arthritis.org for the Arthritis Foundation website.

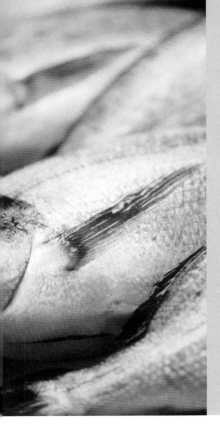

Natural remedies and supplements

For thousands of years, people have turned to natural remedies to relieve their arthritis symptoms. The list of herbal medicines, supplements, and natural preparations seems to grow ever longer, with remarkable claims being made about their efficacy yet very few studies to back them up. Many of these preparations seem to have no effect whatsoever while a few, such as glucosamine and chondroitin, and omega-3 fatty acids, may help alleviate pain and stiffness or reduce inflammation.

Common dietary supplements

People with arthritis are faced with a huge range of products that may or may not help their symptoms. Some may only help certain kinds of arthritis. The choice of products, coupled with often conflicting stories in the press about their safety and effectiveness, can make choosing a supplement daunting.

Glucosamine

An amino sugar found naturally in the body's cartilage, glucosamine may help with joint pain. Several studies suggest that it may be moderately beneficial for the pain and stiffness of osteoarthritis, especially of the knee. Other studies suggest that it may be as effective as ibuprofen for pain relief but the supplements must be taken at least 2 weeks to have an effect.

Glucosamine supplements may be synthetic or include shellfish extracts. The recommended dosage is 750mg of glucosamine, twice a day. It is often combined with chondroitin, and recent research indicates that they are more effective when taken together.

Avoid glucosamine if you have an intolerance or allergy to shellfish, or if you have diabetes.

Chondroitin

Found naturally in the body, this substance is thought to protect cartilage and give it elasticity. Supplements are usually made from the windpipe of cows but do not carry any risk of BSE (a disease in cows linked with a variant of Creutzfeldt–Jakob Disease).

A very large study evaluating chondroitin, chondroitin plus glucosamine, and glucosamine alone showed that in moderate to severe osteoarthritis of the knee, only the combination was effective.

Chondroitin has no toxic side effects, so it may be worth a try. The recommended dosage is 600mg a day. If you experience no benefits within 2–3 months, chondroitin probably does not work for you. If you take warfarin, or have a disorder that affects blood clotting, you should check with your physician before taking chondroitin.

Fish oils

Oily fish, such as salmon, herring, mackerel, tuna, and halibut, as well as cod liver, contain omega-3 fatty acids, such as EPA and DHA. These are important for brain function. More than 20 trials have shown that EPA and DHA inhibit the development of rheumatoid arthritis. They also help boost treatments for depression and lower high blood pressure. The recommended dose is as much as 3g of fish oil supplements a day, which may be as many as 10 or 15 capsules a day. You may experience certain side effects, such as nausea, diarrhea, and nosebleeds. Do not take fish oils if you take anticoagulants such as warfarin. Only take supplements labeled as being free of carcinogens, such as dioxins, that come from pollution in the sea.

Flaxseed oil

Flaxseeds contain the omega-3 fatty acid alpha linolenic acid (ALA). The body may convert this into the fatty acid EPA, which has anti-inflammatory properties. Although flaxseed oil appears to have many benefits, research has not confirmed that it relieves the symptoms of arthritis. However, those who do not want to take fish oils can try flaxseed oil.

Try flaxseed oil in capsule form or add it directly to your food—for example, as a salad dressing. It is a

FLAX
Flax plants (*Linum usitatissimum*) are cultivated for flaxseed oil and linseed oil.

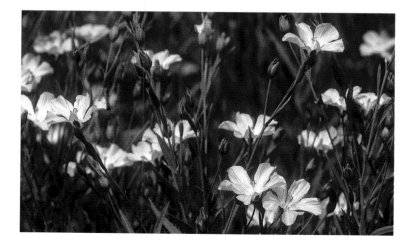

Some evidence suggests that people with pain, morning stiffness, and joint tenderness may derive some benefit from GLA.

natural laxative. However, flaxseed oil may interfere with blood-thinning drugs, such as warfarin, and it should be avoided by women with uterine cancer or hormone-sensitive types of breast cancer.

Collagen

Collagen is a protein found in the body's ligaments and connective tissue. Some scientific evidence suggests that Type II collagen, made from chicken breastbones, may help relieve swollen and tender joints in rheumatoid and juvenile arthritis. Several studies suggest that undenatured collagen (collagen that has not been altered by heat) can help with the mobility and health of joints.

The recommended dosage of undenatured collagen is 60–500 micrograms a day. It has no known interactions with medications, but you should avoid it if you are allergic to chicken or eggs. Consult your physician before trying any Type II collagen supplements.

Cetyl myristolate (CMO)

CMO is a type of fatty acid that is derived from beef tallow. Supplements of CMO have been rumored to help relieve rheumatoid arthritis. However, there is no strong evidence that it works, nor whether it is dangerous or safe, so it should never be substituted for a prescription drug such as methotrexate.

Methylsulfonylmethane

This substance, also known as MSM, is found naturally in the body, as well as in fruits, grains, and vegetables. You can buy it as a supplement to take by mouth or as a gel or lotion to apply externally to affected joints.

MSM has been touted as a remedy for inflammation in arthritis, but there are no independent human studies to support this. It is not known exactly what effects MSM may have in the body. It may interfere with blood-thinning drugs, such as warfarin, and should not be used without informing your physician or rheumatologist first.

MSM was discovered as a byproduct of dimethyl sulfoxide (DMSO), an unpleasant-smelling chemical that is said to relieve inflammation in joints and soft tissues if applied externally to the skin. However, it is not legally available as a supplement and can be highly toxic if it is poor quality. Do not take DMSO without your physician's guidance.

Melatonin

This hormone is produced by the pineal gland in the brain and is involved in regulating the body's sleep–wake cycle. The level of melatonin in the blood is highest at night. It can also be found in some plants and foods. Melatonin supplements are usually synthetic, but some may be derived from animals. Although it is not used as a remedy for arthritis as such, melatonin may help the insomnia associated with chronic or acute pain, although the evidence for this is contradictory.

You should not take large amounts of melatonin supplements because there is evidence that doing so may be linked with depression. Melatonin may also increase the effects of some of the medications that are prescribed to combat anxiety.

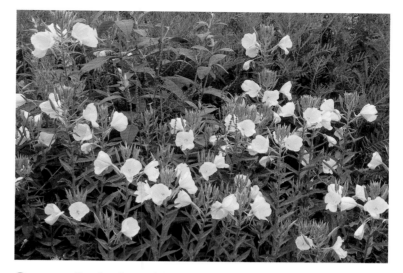

EVENING PRIMROSE
Evening primroses (*Oenothera biennis*) grow wild but are also cultivated for their oil, which contains GLA and has several beneficial properties.

S-adenosyl-L-methione

This substance, also known as SAM-e, occurs naturally in the body, where it plays an important part in chemical reactions. It is claimed to help various conditions, including the pain and stiffness associated with arthritis, and fibromyalgia. Although several trials suggested that SAM-e might have pain-relieving and anti-inflammatory benefits, these benefits have not yet been proven by more rigorous testing methods.

SAM-e comes in tablet form. Many people tolerate it better than NSAIDs. However, high doses can cause gastrointestinal problems and headaches. Avoid SAM-e if you are taking monoamine oxidase inhibitors or antidepressants, or if you have a bipolar disorder or Parkinson's disease. SAM-e can elevate homocysteine levels, so you should also avoid it if you have heart disease.

Gamma linolenic acid

This fatty acid, also known as GLA, is available as a supplement and in the oil of evening primrose. Oils containing GLA have been shown to reduce the inflammation in rheumatoid arthritis. Some evidence suggests that it may relieve some of the pain, morning stiffness, and joint tenderness of rheumatoid arthritis.

The recommended dosage is 1,800mg of GLA supplements a day. You will need to take much more evening primrose oil to receive the same amount of GLA as you would by taking the supplement.

Herbal medicines

Few herbs have been tested for their effect on the symptoms of arthritis, but evidence suggests that some may help relieve inflammation and pain.

Cat's claw

This vine (*Uncaria tomentosa*) grows in the Peruvian Amazon. Its name is derived from the thorns, which are shaped like a cat's claws. The bark of the root is a remedy for inflammation and has been used for boosting immunity, as well as for treating arthritic and gastrointestinal symptoms. Two studies suggest that cat's claw may be useful for treating both osteoarthritis and rheumatoid arthritis.

The recommended dosage is 500–1,000mg of cat's claw, taken as capsules three times a day. Medical herbalists often avoid using it with hormonal drugs, insulin, or vaccines because of potential interactions.

Devil's claw

This shrub from southern Africa is named for its hooked, clawlike seedpods but it is the root that is used. Devil's claw contains harpagoside, shown in two trials to reduce inflammation and pain.

You can take devil's claw as a capsule or as a tincture or tea. It may interfere with warfarin or drugs used for irregular heartbeats and diabetes. Check with your physician first if you have gallstones or gastric or duodenal ulcers. Avoid it if you are pregnant or are taking NSAIDs (see p.72).

DEVIL'S CLAW
The root of devil's claw (*Harpagophytum procumbens*) is a traditional remedy for relieving pain and inflammation.

Cayenne

Also known as paprika, chili pepper, or red pepper, cayenne (*Capsicum frutescens*) is a remedy for various conditions, including arthritic pain and stomach upsets. Capsaicin, the active ingredient of cayenne, stimulates the release of endorphins, which are the body's own pain relievers. A randomized, placebo-controlled trial showed that it is effective in relieving osteoarthritic and rheumatoid arthritic pain. Many people suffering from arthritis regularly rub capsaicin cream onto their affected joints.

You should avoid putting the cream on broken or irritated skin. Wash your hands thoroughly after use and before touching your eyes. Eating too much cayenne can be dangerous because it may raise your body temperature.

Boswellia

This herb (*Boswellia thurifera*), which produces the frankincense resin, is used in Chinese and Ayurvedic medicine for the relief of arthritic pain. A few studies suggest that boswellia may help relieve the inflammation of arthritis, especially when boswellia is combined with an Indian herb called ashwagandha. However, there is little scientific evidence to confirm that it is safe. The recommended dosage is 150mg of boswellia extract, taken three times a day.

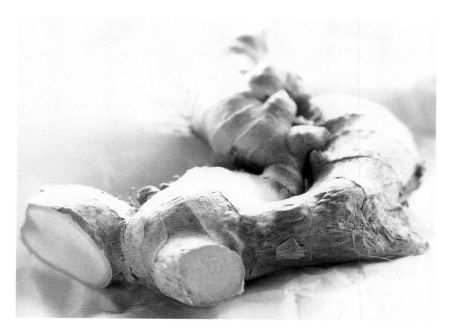

Ginger

Ginger root is a traditional remedy for digestive disorders, such as nausea, and arthritic pain. One trial showed that ginger eased the pain of osteoarthritis. It may help relieve pain and inflammation because it seems to block the action of chemicals in the body, such as leukotrienes, that cause pain and swelling.

Cook with ginger regularly but avoid it if you are taking blood thinning drugs, such as warfarin, or if you have gallstones, diabetes, or heart problems—unless your physician approves.

Bromelain

This protein-digesting enzyme is extracted from the pineapple plant (*Ananas comosus*). Several trials suggest it is an anti-inflammatory and may help with pain relief in arthritis. The recommended dosage is 400–600mg of bromelain extract, taken in capsules three times a day. You should avoid it during pregnancy or while breastfeeding. It may interfere with blood-thinning drugs such as warfarin and large doses may cause stomach upsets.

Turmeric

A spice traditionally used in cooking, turmeric (**Curcuma longa**) has been used in traditional Chinese and Ayurvedic medicine to ease inflammation and pain in arthritis. Small studies suggest that it has an effect when used in combination with other supplements, but there is no scientific evidence that it works alone. High doses of turmeric may

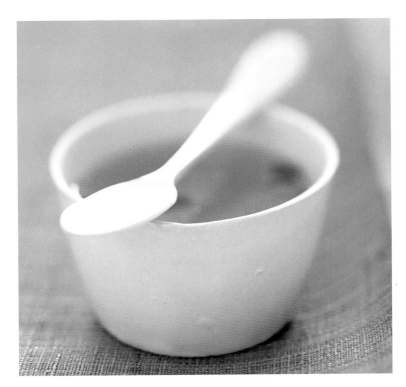

GREEN TEA
Regular consumption of green tea may protect against certain cancers, dental decay, heart disease, kidney stones, and bacterial infections.

(*Hypericum perforatum*) can ease the symptoms of mild to moderate depression, but there is no evidence that it eases the symptoms of arthritis, such as inflammation. Check with your physician before taking St. John's wort because it may interfere with certain medicines and may cause side effects, such as sensitivity to sunlight, insomnia, and gastrointestinal problems. Do not take this if you are taking prescription antidepressants.

Green Tea
Drinking green tea may contribute to your general health because of the antioxidants it contains. As yet, there is no firm evidence that green tea directly helps relieve arthritis symptoms, although research studies on animals are showing promise.

Burdock
The root of burdock (*Arctium lappa*) is touted for removing waste material from inflamed joints and has been used for many conditions, including arthritis. However, no convincing scientific evidence exists to show that it is effective.

If you suffer from diabetes, always check with your physician before taking it. Burdock may also affect oral contraceptives, hormone replacement therapy (HRT), and blood-thinning drugs such as warfarin or heparin.

act as a blood thinner and may also cause gastrointestinal upsets. Therefore, you should avoid turmeric if you have gallstones or take blood thinners.

Valerian
A couple of scientific trials suggest that valerian may help prevent insomnia and relieve anxiety, and therefore may be useful for those with chronic or acute pain. Do not take valerian with sedatives or hypnotic drugs. Excess valerian may cause serious side effects.

St. John's Wort
There is good evidence to suggest that a supplement made from the leaves and stem of St. John's wort

Trace minerals

You should be able to receive all the trace minerals you need from a balanced diet. However, people with various forms of arthritis may benefit from taking extra mineral supplements.

Copper

People who take copper as a supplement or wear it against their skin as a bracelet believe it can relieve pain and inflammation. However, there is no convincing evidence of this. You can get all the copper you need from a daily multivitamin supplement.

Taking too much copper in supplement form may lead to an overdose, which can be very dangerous or even fatal. Do not wear a magnetic copper bracelet if you are pregnant, have a medical device such as a pacemaker, or are using medication patches.

Selenium

Selenium is a trace mineral that is essential in small amounts for your health. Found in plants, meat, and seafoods, it may be helpful in a number of serious diseases, including cancer, heart disease, and arthritis. Some studies have found lower levels of selenium in people with rheumatoid arthritis. The recommended dose is 50–200 micrograms; you should be able to get all you need in a multivitamin. Too much selenium can be toxic.

Manganese

Manganese is a trace mineral that is essential for health. It is found in leafy vegetables, nuts, teas, and whole grains. There is no evidence that manganese supplements have any effect on arthritis but selenium may help keep bones healthy. It may also affect the absorption of certain drugs, such as antacids, laxatives, and tetracyclines. In addition, people with liver failure should avoid it.

Homeopathic medicines

A homeopath experienced in treating arthritis may suggest one of the following.

Rhus toxicodendron

Rhus tox, which is made from poison ivy, may help with the morning stiffness that is typical of osteoarthritis.

Apis mellifica

Apis mellifica is believed by homeopaths to relieve the hot, swollen, and tender joints that are common in rheumatoid arthritis.

Causticum

Causticum, which is derived from a potassium compound, may help people who have joints that seem to be very sensitive to the weather.

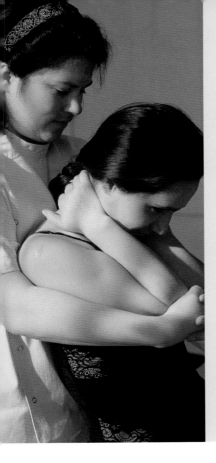

Bodywork therapies

The healing power of touch has been an important part of healthcare since antiquity. Manipulation and bodywork practices, such as massage, chiropractic, and osteopathy, are among the more respected and trustworthy of the complementary therapies. In experienced hands, they can ease restrictions, alleviate pain, and restore lost function. At their heart, they are holistic practices that seek to rebalance the body's equilibrium and reestablish the integrated nature of the musculoskeletal system.

Osteopathy, like chiropractic, focuses on the spine and joints and hinges on the belief that the body has the ability to heal itself.

Chiropractic

Chiropractic is a therapy that focuses on the relationship between the structure of the body, mainly the spine, and overall well-being. Aspects of chiropractic have existed for thousands of years, but the modern profession was founded in 1895 by Daniel David Palmer, a Canadian who believed that the body has its own natural healing ability that is controlled by the nervous system.

The spine and other joints, such as those linking the spine and pelvis, may "go out of alignment" according to chiropractic beliefs.

Misalignments, or subluxations, of the spine disrupt the nervous system and lead to various complaints and diseases.

Chiropractic has different branches, such as McTimoney chiropractic, but they all highlight the fundamental link between the nervous system and overall health. Chiropractors can perform X-rays and prescribe some medications but are not medical doctors.

Chiropractors believe the therapy can help a wide range of conditions, from migraines and back pain to irritable bowel syndrome and asthma. Some evidence suggests that chiropractic can ease acute or chronic lower back pain, but no evidence that it helps with arthritis.

■ **WHAT TO EXPECT AT A CHIROPRACTIC SESSION** Chiropractors will usually begin by discussing your overall health and medical history. They may take X–rays of your spine and will physically examine you, probably in just your underwear, as you sit or lie down.

Chiropractors use a range of different manipulation techniques known as adjustments. Some of these are sharp, jerky movements (known as "high-velocity thrusts") on different parts of the body. You will sometimes hear popping or cracking noises, which are simply the release of tiny air bubbles in the fluid at the surface of a joint. Usually, you will require more than one treatment.

■ **SAFETY ISSUES** Manipulation of inflamed joints and overexposure to X–rays should be avoided. Consult your physician first if you have osteoporosis, bleeding problems, or a malignant or inflammatory spinal disease.

Osteopathy

Osteopathy, like chiropractic, focuses on the spine and joints, and hinges on the belief that the body has the ability to heal itself. It was pioneered by American doctor Andrew Taylor Still in 1874. Osteopaths work on the premise that misalignments of the skeleton can affect the fluids of the body and lead to a range of conditions, including arthritis.

Osteopaths use manipulation techniques, such as high-velocity thrusts, combined with slightly gentler maneuvers, including soft-tissue massage, to correct misalignments and let the body heal itself. Osteopaths treat children as well as adults.

Osteopaths undergo a similar amount of training as medical physicians and practice as physicians with an emphasis on manipulation and massage. An osteopath's degree is "DO"—doctor of osteopathy—rather than "MD."

Osteopathy is used for various conditions, including arthritis, sports injuries, sciatica, and frozen shoulder. The overall emphasis is on improving mobility, so an osteopath may give you advice on exercise and posture. Scientific evidence indicates that osteopathy can help lower back pain.

■ **WHAT TO EXPECT AT AN OSTEOPATHY SESSION** The osteopath will start by taking your full medical history. You will need to remove some of your clothes to allow the osteopath to assess the biomechanics of your body, including posture, and to look for excessive strains or weaknesses. Many osteopaths provide primary care services as well as bodywork therapies.

■ **SAFETY ISSUES** The same as for chiropractic (see above).

SOFT-TISSUE MASSAGE

Massage in its various forms can relieve arthritis symptoms such as pain, stiffness, tension, and immobility. The treatment increases blood flow to the muscles to reduce tension, thereby relieving pain and encouraging mobility. Some forms of massage use oils or special instruments to add to the therapeutic effect.

THERAPY	WHAT IS IT GOOD FOR?
Swedish massage Involves kneading (petrissage) or rhythmic stroking (effleurage) of muscles and soft tissues; may include oils or electrical stimulation devices.	Reduces general stiffness and releases tension. May help rheumatoid arthritis, osteoarthritis, fibromyalgia.
Chair massage Manipulation in a specially designed chair that bends your body to improve the practitioner's access to your tense joints.	Neck and back joint pain, fibromyalgia, and arthritis pain —as long as you can sit comfortably in the chair.
Myofascial release Slow, gentle manipulation of your fascia—the thin tissues surrounding muscles—to stretch your tense tissues and relieve pain and stress.	Fibromyalgia and general stress relief associated with any chronic illness.
Deep tissue massage Releases tension in deeper layers of soft tissue than Swedish massage, with manipulation across the grain of your muscle; it also may break up scar tissue within the soft tissues.	General arthritis. It is especially good for back pain associated with arthritis.

Massage

Massage is one of the oldest forms of complementary therapy and dates back at least as far as ancient Egypt. Modern massage, which is sometimes also known as Swedish massage, was developed in the 19th century by a Swede called Per Henrik Ling. Now there are many different kinds, including massage techniques that are gentler than Ling's quite vigorous methods. There are various soft-tissue massage techniques (see left), some of which may also use aromatherapy oils (see p.124).

Massage is used for a wide range of conditions, from back pain and fibromylagia, to irritable bowel syndrome, headaches, and general stress relief, and the evidence to support its use is relatively positive.

■ **WHAT TO EXPECT AT A MASSAGE SESSION** You will usually have to take off some of your clothes before the massage starts. The therapist will use a variety of rubbing, stroking, pressing, or kneading techniques that may be vigorous and stimulating, or gentle and relaxing, or a combination of both. During the massage, the therapist may use creams, oils, or talcum powder.

■ **SAFETY ISSUES** Anyone who is suffering from deep vein thrombosis, burns, skin diseases or infections, open wounds, osteoporosis, or bone fractures should seek medical advice before receiving a massage.

Rolfing

Rolfing is a deep pressure form of massage that was developed in the 1950s by Dr. Ida Rolf, who believed that releasing muscle tension would lead to overall health. Rolfing is also referred to as "structural integration" and is used for general stress relief, headaches, and back pain. However, there is no strong evidence that it works.

■ **WHAT TO EXPECT AT A ROLFING SESSION**
There are similarities with other forms of massage, but the techniques are often more forceful and probing.

■ **SAFETY ISSUES** Damage may be caused to those with rheumatoid arthritis or other inflammatory joint disorders. Avoid any painful or uncomfortable massage if you have a flare-up in your condition. (See also Massage, opposite.)

Reiki

Reiki is a touch therapy that originated in Japan at the start of the 20th century. It is based on the idea that good health comes from a balanced "energy flow" in the body. Reiki in Japanese translates as "universal energy" and the therapist aims to use this universal energy to improve your personal energy flow. Reiki is used as a general therapy to ease stress or promote relaxation, but there is no scientific evidence that it works.

■ **WHAT TO EXPECT AT A REIKI SESSION**
You sit or lie down but do not usually need to remove any clothes. The therapist then lays both hands gently on different parts of your body.

■ **SAFETY ISSUES** There are no known safety issues.

Acupuncture

Acupuncture is perhaps the most ancient of all the complementary therapies; Chinese texts refer to it from the first century BC, but it is probably even older than that.

Acupuncture is based on the belief that good health comes from a perfect balance between two opposites—*yin* and *yang*. Diseases or health complaints occur because of an imbalance between *yin* and *yang*, which upsets the flow of the body's vital energy, known as *qi* (pronounced "chee"). This energy moves through the body along meridians, a network of 12 pathways that feature more than 350 acupoints.

Acupuncturists insert tiny needles into specific acupoints to adjust the flow of *qi* and rebalance the *yin* and *yang*. Practitioners of acupressure, or a similar therapy called shiatsu, use their fingers and hands instead of needles.

ACUPUNCTURE TREATMENT
An acupuncturist inserts a needle into the tissue just below the skin. The treatment may require the acupuncturist to insert needles into several acupoints.

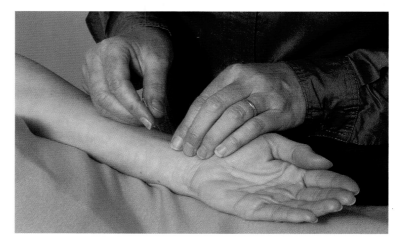

Acupuncture is reimbursed by some health insurance companies, and many pain clinics offer it alongside conventional treatments.

Acupuncture can be used for many conditions, including pain from osteoarthritis, fibromyalgia, nausea, headache, depression, and back pain. However, the evidence for its effectiveness is mixed and depends on the condition: there is strong evidence for relief of dental pain and nausea, promising evidence for fibromyalgia, but conflicting evidence for treating back pain and osteoarthritis. Nevertheless, acupuncture has been shown to cause the brain to release endorphins (chemicals that may ease pain).

■ **WHAT TO EXPECT AT AN ACUPUNCTURE SESSION** In the first session, the acupuncturist will discuss your health complaint and take your full medical history before deciding on treatment.

The acupuncturist inserts a series of long, thin, disposable needles just under the surface of the skin at various acupoints that may be on the face and scalp. This usually does not hurt, although some people may experience a little discomfort, such as a tingling sensation at the site of the needles. The needles are left in for a few seconds or up to 20 minutes.

■ **SAFETY ISSUES** The needles should be used only once. People with a severe bleeding disorder should not receive acupuncture.

ESSENTIAL OILS

Aromatherapy oils, also known as essential oils, are often used in massage. They come from plant essences, have unique properties, and may be applied directly to the skin in a carrier oil, inhaled with steam, or used to scent a room via a diffuser. The evidence of their effectiveness is inconclusive, although some oils may help anxiety, relieve insomnia, or combat fungal infections.

OIL	WHAT IS IT GOOD FOR?
Lavender	General relaxation. Aid for insomnia, stress, or anxiety.
Marjoram, Spanish	To promote relaxation and ease muscle fatigue.
Rosemary	To reduce pain and swelling and improve circulation.
Thyme	To ease joint pain.
Ylang Ylang	For anxiety and insomnia.
Chamomile	To ease muscle and rheumatic pain and promote relaxation.

Aromatherapy

Aromatherapy is said to help increase vitality, improve well-being, and restore health. Its unique oils have been used for various ailments (see left).

Aromatherapy is easy to use, making it a good candidate for self-treatment at home. You can massage the oils into your skin, inhale them, or add them to a bath. However, you will get the best treatment from a professional aromatherapist.

■ **WHAT TO EXPECT AT AN AROMATHERAPY SESSION** You will be asked about your past and present state of health, diet, and lifestyle. The therapist will select suitable oils, ask you to remove some of your clothes, and then give you a massage using the oils.

■ **SAFETY ISSUES** Check with your physician before using any essential oils in the first three months of pregnancy. Always check with your children's pediatrician before using oils on children. Large quantities of any oil may be dangerous and they should never be directly ingested.

Reflexology

Reflexology is a therapy that focuses on the feet and sometimes the hands. The modern form of reflexology was developed in the early 20th century by William Fitzgerald, an American ear, nose, and throat specialist.

The idea is that zones on the soles of the feet or palms of the hands reflect corresponding organs and parts of the body. By massaging the zones in a selective way, a reflexologist can remove blockages of energy, thereby easing or even curing various ailments.

Reflexology may benefit many disorders, but is most often used for stress relief, arthritis, irritable bowel syndrome, headaches, and premenstrual problems. The

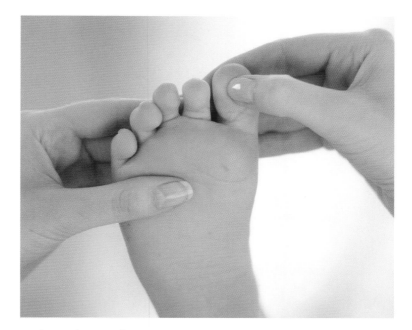

REFLEXOLOGY MASSAGE
A reflexologist uses thumb or finger pressure to massage particular areas of the feet.

evidence for its effectiveness is not conclusive although some evidence suggests it can help headaches and premenstrual problems.

■ **WHAT TO EXPECT AT A REFLEXOLOGY SESSION** After giving your detailed medical history, you will need to take off your shoes and socks and may either sit or lie down. By applying finger and thumb pressure, the reflexologist will massage selected areas of your feet, and occasionally your hands.

Treatment does not usually feel ticklish—in fact, most people find it very relaxing, although some of the strokes can be quite firm and intense. You can expect to have several sessions, usually one a week for 6 weeks.

■ **SAFETY ISSUES** People with bone or joint problems in the feet should be treated with extra care.

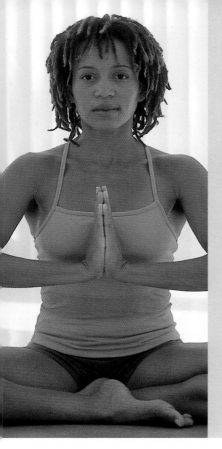

Movement therapies

Keeping mobile is very important for people with arthritis. When your joints are stiff or sore, it is often tempting to avoid using them, but this can become a downward spiral, leading to greater pain and disability. Movement therapies, such as yoga, tai chi, and the Alexander Technique, help you learn new ways of holding, stretching, and moving your body. These changes will bring about improvements to your posture that might not only ease symptoms but also lead to an overall sensation of well-being.

Osteopaths and chiropractors often recommend Pilates to people who suffer from back problems because it focuses on core strength, which involves toning and strengthening the abdomen.

Yoga

The word "yoga" comes from the Sanskrit "yuj," which means to yoke, or unite. The practice of yoga focuses on unifying the mind, body, and spirit in a way that is claimed to bring good health and a relaxed state of mind.

In the West, the most commonly practiced type of yoga is hatha yoga, which is based on poses (asanas), meditation, and breath control (pranayama). Yoga teachers will show you how to stretch and hold your body in the different poses and and how to practice breathing and meditation.

■ **WHO IS YOGA SUITABLE FOR?** Yoga may be suitable for everyone, young or old and whether or not you have arthritis. If yoga suits you, be prepared to practice it regularly as part of an ongoing, long-term commitment.

■ **HOW MIGHT YOGA HELP ME?** Yoga has been shown to improve mood and well-being. Specifically, it may help those with high blood pressure and joint stiffness. One study found that it eased the symptoms of rheumatoid arthritis.

■ **SAFETY ISSUES** Don't overextend yourself and do try to find a qualified instructor who can teach yoga to people with arthritis.

Pilates

This technique focuses on a series of exercises designed to strengthen the body, improve flexibility, and help with overall posture. It also involves concentration and learning to breathe in a controlled, supposedly beneficial way. The exercises may be carried out on mats at home or in a class, or by using special apparatus in a Pilates studio. There are several different forms, each based on the exercises developed by Joseph Pilates in the early 1920s in Germany.

■ **WHO IS PILATES SUITABLE FOR?** Pilates is suitable for anyone, including the elderly, pregnant women, and people with arthritis. It is important to choose the right level for your needs.

■ **HOW MIGHT PILATES HELP ME?**
Osteopaths and chiropractors often recommend Pilates to people who suffer from back problems because it focuses on core strength, which involves toning and strengthening the abdomen.

Pilates can also help you correctly align your pelvis and spine. The movements are very gentle and slow, although they can become much more difficult as you progress and develop strength. One study shows that it may help joint mobility, but there is no research into its effects on arthritis.

■ **SAFETY ISSUES** Pilates is relatively gentle and should not present any safety concerns. As with all forms of exercise, avoid movements that feel painful, particularly if you have inflamed joints.

PRACTICAL TIPS

SAFETY ISSUES

In all movement therapies, make sure you:

● Don't overextend yourself.

● Only move your body and limbs within a range that is comfortable for you—your comfort zone. There is no place for the notion of "no pain, no gain."

● Stop at once If any movement feels painful or uncomfortable.

● Tell your instructor, before you begin a class, that you have arthritis and explain how you are affected by it.

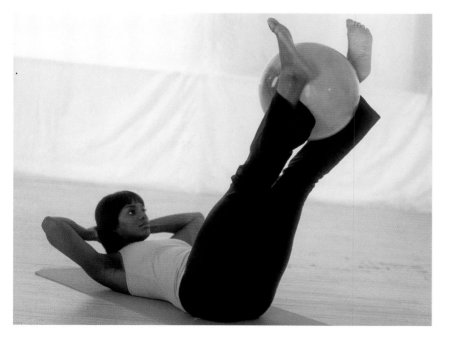

PRACTICING PILATES
Special equipment is not essential for practicing Pilates at home, although a mat, a rolled-up towel, and a sizeable ball are useful.

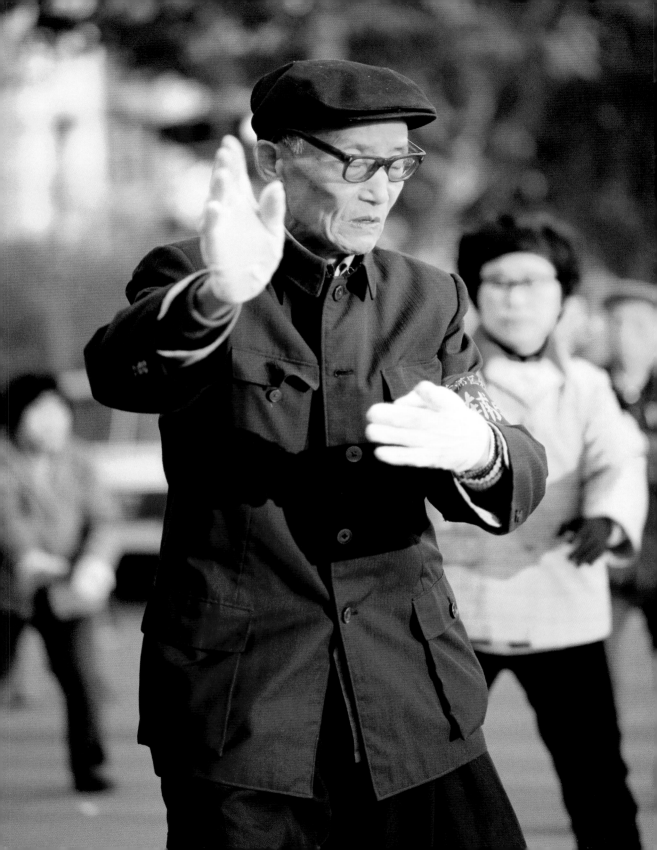

Tai chi

Tai chi is a system of movements and postures with roots in both martial arts and ancient Chinese philosophy. It is designed to improve strength and flexibility and promote overall well-being through body harmony. Like acupuncture (see p.117), tai chi embodies the principle that disharmony between the fundamental forces of *yin* and *yang* leads to health complaints, including pain and disease.

Tai chi is taught in small classes in which certain slow movements are combined with deep breathing and concentration. If tai chi suits you, be prepared to practice it for a short time each day and to make it a lifelong commitment.

■ **WHO IS TAI CHI SUITABLE FOR?** Tai chi is suitable for everyone, including elderly people and people with arthritis.

■ **HOW MIGHT TAI CHI HELP ME?** Tai chi is an easy technique to learn, can relieve pain and stress, and brings inner peace. It helps align your spine and takes many of your joints through their normal range of movement.

Tai chi has been shown to help with developing balance and strength in a way that improves confidence and reduces falls in elderly people. It has also helped relieve depression and fatigue, and improve the function of the heart and lungs of elderly people.

A trial of elderly women with osteoarthritis of the knee also showed a benefit from learning tai chi.

■ **SAFETY ISSUES** Tai chi is a relatively gentle therapy, with no known health or safety concerns.

Qi gong

Qi gong is a traditional Chinese technique that combines meditation and movement to build stamina and ease the stress of chronic conditions.

■ **WHO IS QI GONG SUITABLE FOR?** Like tai chi, Qi gong is suitable for everyone, including elderly people and people with arthritis.

■ **HOW MIGHT QI GONG HELP ME?** Qi gong is used in traditional

Tai chi is taught in small classes in which certain slow movements are combined with deep breathing and concentration.

TAI CHI OUTDOORS
Each day, Chinese people gather outdoors, in the park or in the street, to practice the sequences of tai chi.

Q&A

"Will the movements of tai chi help me to fight my arthritis?"

No. Try not to think in terms of "fighting" your disease—you are not being "attacked," nor do you have to "conquer" your condition. Although tai chi has its roots in martial arts, its movements are graceful, not aggressive. They will encourage you to focus your physical and mental energies in a way that helps you protect your health.

Chinese medicine for many medical conditions. Some evidence suggests that Qi gong may help people with high blood pressure, although the research is limited.

It is possible that Qi gong may be an aid to relaxation, which could in theory help with the management of pain or stress, but there is no hard scientific evidence to support this.

■ **SAFETY ISSUES** Qi gong is thought to be safe. Rarely, the symptoms of people with psychiatric conditions may get worse. If you have a psychiatric disorder, speak to your physician before trying Qi gong.

CORRECTING BAD POSTURE
A practitioner of the Alexander Technique can help you undo your postural bad habits and learn new ways of sitting and standing that avoid tension.

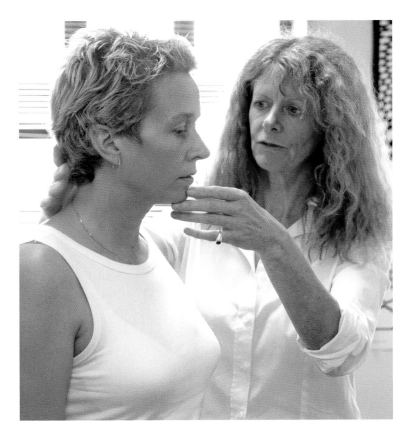

Alexander Technique

The Alexander Technique is a way of learning to correctly hold and move your body so that you can improve your posture, balance, and coordination. Australian actor Frederick Alexander developed the technique at the start of the 20th century after he suffered problems with his voice.

After observing himself in a mirror, he realized that he was holding his neck in a tense position and wondered if this was the root of his trouble. He gradually worked on solving the problem by devising a series of movements that altered the way he held his head, neck, and spine.

The Alexander Technique is often taught in drama schools as a way of helping students learn to move and use their bodies freely, but it is also used to help with voice problems. The technique is also used by some athletes.

■ **HOW MIGHT THE ALEXANDER TECHNIQUE HELP ME?** The technique is based on the idea that the head, neck, and spine play a crucial role in the overall flexibility and health of the body. Over the years, you have probably developed awkward ways of sitting, standing, and moving. You unconsciously tense up with anxiety or stress and adopt poor postures that affect the way you move your body.

Alexander teachers work with people on a one-on-one basis and gently use their hands to show you how to correct postural problems and to learn to use your body in the most "natural" way.

The technique has been shown to benefit people with respiratory problems and back pain, and to work on the body's autonomic nervous system to help relieve stress and anxiety.

■ **SAFETY ISSUES** There are no known safety issues.

Feldenkrais method

This therapy is like the Alexander Technique in that it teaches you patterns of movement that help ease your health complaints and maximize your flexibility. The method was developed by Israeli physicist Moshe Feldenkrais after he suffered a serious knee injury.

In a small class, known as Awareness Through Movement, you learn a series of gentle movements that you can do while sitting, standing, or lying down. Alternatively, you can have one-to-one consultations, known as Functional Integration, in which the teacher uses his or her hands to guide you directly. You may also receive a massage.

■ **HOW MIGHT THE FELDENKRAIS METHOD HELP ME?** People may learn the Feldenkrais Method for many reasons, such as rehabilitation after an accident, alleviating anxiety and stress, or relieving pain. There is

evidence that it may have mild benefits for low back pain, and also for shoulder and neck pain.

■ **SAFETY ISSUES** There are no known safety issues, but if you have suffered an injury or are recovering from surgery, consult your physician first.

Trager approach

Proponents of the Trager Approach believe that ill-health and stress stem from the unconscious mind. The method was developed in America by Milton Trager, a boxer turned physician who realized that a range of movements and touch techniques can change unhealthy mental and physical habits.

A session of Trager work will involve lying on a padded table in a semimeditative state while the therapist moves your body in certain ways, using rocking, gentle shaking, or stretching techniques.

You can also practice a series of mental exercises, known as "Mentastics," at home. One example involves you shifting the way you hold your weight in order to maintain a "freer" body.

■ **HOW MIGHT THE TRAGER APPROACH HELP ME?** Very little research exists, and this method is rarely used or available. One study has shown that the Trager Approach may benefit people with back pain.

■ **SAFETY ISSUES** There are no known safety issues.

Alexander teachers work with people on a one-to-one basis and gently use their hands to show you how to correct postural problems and to learn to use your body in the most "natural" way.

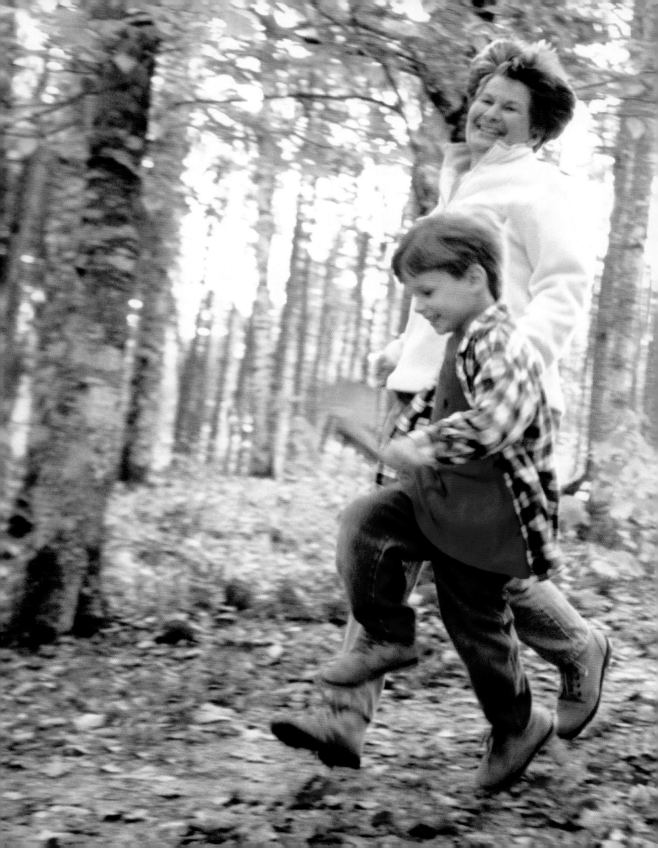

Living with arthritis

If you have been diagnosed with arthritis you will need to make changes to the way you live your life. How extensive those changes become will depend on the type of arthritis you have and how it is affecting you. People with a mild condition may only need to make minor adjustments, while those who are affected more severely may find that there are many challenges to address.

Occupational therapists, physical therapists, and many other specialists can provide you with a great deal of advice and guidance to help you manage your arthritis and deal with issues that arise in everyday life. Such issues include the impact of arthritis on your work, domestic activities, driving, family life, and personal relationships.

One aspect of arthritis that can be hard is not knowing how long it is going to last or when it is going to flare up into an episode of pain, inflammation, and swelling. Coping with these episodes can be stressful, so it is good to learn and practice techniques that not only help you get through the pain and stress but also protect your joints from potential damage.

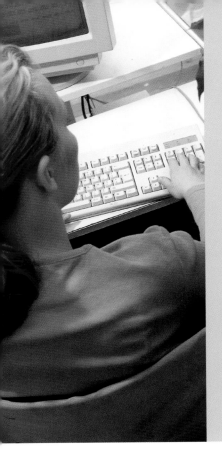

Day-to-day living

The pain, stiffness, and other symptoms of your arthritis can have a profound impact on the way you go about your day-to-day living. Your work may be compromised and your domestic life may become a daily challenge. But there is no reason to despair because there are many different sources of help available to you. Laws protect your rights at work, occupational therapists can help you solve your practical problems, and friends and family will give you all the support you need. For those who cherish their independence, a host of assistive devices and energy-saving tips are available to make your life much easier.

It is important to identify and resolve potential problems as early as possible.

Working

If you are diagnosed with arthritis one of your first concerns may be how the condition will affect your job or your chances of getting one. Questions may concern short- and long-term finances, your manager's reaction, or how you will perform some aspects of your job.

Don't panic. Various people and organizations can help if you are having difficulties (see p.135). In the US, legislation gives you certain rights. If, for example, you have rheumatoid arthritis, you can't be laid off because of your condition. The Americans with Disabilities Act (1990) states that your employer must make reasonable accommodations to your current job or consider you for suitable vacancies within the company. However, you must educate yourself regarding your rights under the Occupational Safety and Health Act (1970) and the ADA Accessibility Guidelines for Buildings and Facilities (1991, amended 2002).

Modifying the workplace
If arthritis does not compromise your job excessively and your manager wants you to stay, it is important to identify and resolve

potential problems as early as possible. If you can't solve them, seek independent advice (see Who can help, right).

Under the law, your place of employment should be accessible to anyone with a disability. Your employer also has a duty to make "reasonable accommodations" that will not cause disproportionate disruption and that are affordable to the business. These include:

• Changes to your working environment, such as ergonomic changes to your work station, an allocated parking space, and suitable building alterations.

• Changes to your job description.

• Change to your timetable, such as new working hours, flexible working, and change of shifts.

• The purchase of modified equipment and assistive devices, such as a chunky pen or a dictaphone if writing is difficult.

• A job coach to train you in the tasks required to perform a job.

Returning to work

If you have to take a significant amount of time off because of arthritis—for surgery, for example—a successful return can depend on a number of factors, including a discussion with your employer before you leave; the nature of your job; the severity of your condition; and how long you have been away.

Tell your employer—both your boss and the human resources

department—about your arthritis and discuss the changes you will need. Suggest a gradual return and ask for a regular review. If you can only manage a part-time job, estimate the minimum salary you need to live on. Your occupational therapist can advise you.

WHO CAN HELP?

You and your manager may be able to solve the workplace problems yourselves. If you need extra help, the following people and organizations can give you advice, information, and/or practical help about working with arthritis. You need to get as much information and advice as possible to help you cope and to make an informed decision about your future.

PROFESSIONAL	WHAT'S AVAILABLE
Occupational health provider	Ask to be referred for an occupational health assessment. Some companies and organizations have their own doctors and nurses; a few also employ counselors, physical therapists, and occupational therapists, so it is worth asking for an appointment with one of them.
Human resources representative	Your company's human resources department, especially the benefits manager, will help you determine which ones might work for you, for example, the Family and Medical Leave Act (FMLA, 1993)
Union representative	Depending on the nature of your employment, your best source of information may be your union representative.
Healthcare professional (physician, rheumatologist, etc.)	Medical advice and information.
Rheumatology occupational therapist	Advice and information on work issues. Some may offer an enhanced service, such as performing a work assessment or a work report with recommendations.

Household chores

The bending, lifting, pushing, gripping, and carrying that are involved in doing housework can take their toll on sore and aching joints and leave you with little energy to spare for more enjoyable leisure activities.

Think of easier ways of doing things. Try sitting while you are preparing food. Use energy-saving equipment, such as a microwave or electric can opener. Well-designed tools will require less effort to use and are less stressful for your joints. A good example is the chunky grip on hand tools, such a chopping knife and a screwdriver, or on lever door handles and faucets. If you have painful wrists or knees, wear a supportive splint.

■ **CLEANING** Try keeping an upright posture, bending your knees rather than your back, and don't try to clean the whole house at one time! A lightweight, upright vacuum cleaner may be easier to use than a canister model. Check that you can grip the handle, operate the controls, and change the bags easily before you buy one. Ask someone to carry the vacuum cleaner upstairs for you or keep another one up there permanently.

Bending to pick items off the floor can be difficult. A pick-up stick or long-handled dustpan and brush can be useful. To save on trips upstairs when neatening up, collect items in a basket at the bottom of the stairs and take them all up at one time.

■ **LAUNDRY** Front-loading washing machines and driers are easier to reach if mounted on a firm base. If you prefer hanging clothes out on a line to dry, use clothespins rather than squeeze-open clips. If you find reaching up difficult, try using a clothesline and prop it up with a forked stick. The line can be

COPING WITH HOUSEWORK

Cleaning, tidying, making meals, doing the laundry, ironing, and all those other chores that constitute household work can be tiring at the best of times. There are a number of tips that will conserve your energy, protect your joints, and generally make your life much easier.

TIP	ACTIVITY
Plan ahead	Make a list of household jobs and plan to do a little over several days, rather than all at once. Plan rest days and make a list of potential helpers.
Pace yourself	Take regular breaks when doing housework. Be systematic and avoid unnecessary trips around the house and upstairs.
Posture and position	Keep a relaxed upright posture, bending from the knees rather than the back. Change position often and avoid gripping things tightly for long periods—for example, when polishing or scouring pots.
Get help	Ask family or friends to help with heavier tasks. You may be able to pay someone to do the cleaning for you.
Storage	Store items that you often use at the front of cabinets at chest height. Throw away old articles that you no longer use and keep cabinets uncluttered.

lowered to allow you to peg on the clothes and then raised to dry.

When ironing, wear a wrist support, use a lightweight iron, and sit on a stool (see p.176). Iron a little at a time and if you have room, leave the board standing. Many synthetic fabrics do not need to be ironed at all.

■ **MAKING BEDS** Stretchy man-made fabrics with fitted sheets and lightweight comforters may be easier to manage. Velcro fastenings on covers are easier on arthritic hands than snaps.

■ **MEAL PREPARATION** If you cook often and you can afford them, buy lightweight power tools to stir, chop, grate, and whisk food. Use a knife and vegetable peeler with a chunky grip.

Chose appliances, such as a stove and microwave, that you can reach into safely and that feature easy-to-operate controls. Use lightweight pans for cooking, preferably with two handles.

To avoid the strain on your joints of having to pick up a heavy pan of water, steam or microwave vegetables. If you use a saucepan, put a frying basket in the pan. When the vegetables are done you can remove the basket and leave the pan and hot water to cool. Alternatively, use a slotted spoon.

If you do not eat in the kitchen, a cart can be helpful to take food through to another room. Keep some frozen meals available for "bad days."

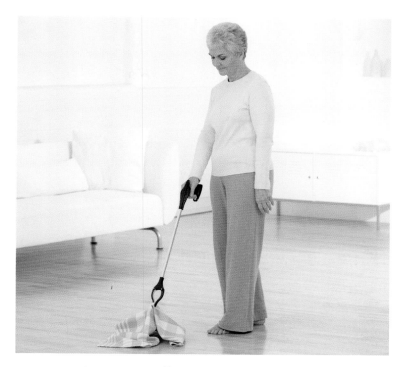

■ **WASHING UP** Most items will go in a dishwasher, although it will be most effective if you promptly rinse off any food before you put it in the diswasher. If you wash and dry by hand, rest the pans either in the sink or on the drain board.

■ **SHOPPING** Internet shopping and home-delivery services have made shopping easier for many people. Most supermarkets will pack groceries and take them to your car. Some discount stores also have clip-on carts for wheelchairs. Facilitated mobility within the store and nearby disabled parking lots are available in most areas.

■ **IN THE WORKSHOP AND GARDEN** By adapting the ideas mentioned above, you can successfully garden and carry out maintenance tasks.

PICK-UP TOOL
You can avoid the pain of bending down to pick things up off the floor if you use a pick-up tool.

SOLVING EVERYDAY PROBLEMS

Many assistive devices are either based on common sense or are the result of ingenious solutions. They are all derived from tried-and-tested ways of helping you solve manual problems and accomplish everyday activities that are taken for granted for people who do not have arthritis.

ACTIVITY	PROBLEM	SOLUTION
Writing	Weak grip because of painful wrist and fingers.	Use a pen with a chunky, rubber grip and try to relax your grip on the pen as you write.
Peeling potatoes	Gripping and turning the peeler.	Choose a wide-handled peeler (available in most cooking stores).
Washing and drying feet, neck, and back	Reaching becomes difficult due to pain.	Wash with a long-handled sponge. Dry with a lightweight towel that has hand loops. Wear a terrycloth bathrobe.
Turning a key	Gripping and turning a key.	Fit a handle to your key to give you better leverage.
Picking up things from the floor	Reaching down.	Use a pick-up tool (see p.137).

Splints

Wearing a splint can support and protect unstable and painful joints in your body, such as the wrists, hands, fingers, knees, and ankles. Splints can help you walk, grip, handle objects, and may ease pain and swelling. You can either buy a standard version at a pharmacy or medical supply store or you can request a custom-made splint from your occupational therapist or physical therapist.

Home modifications

You may wish to modify your home in order to improve your ability to get around. For example, if you have arthritis in your hips, knees, or ankles, you may have difficulty rising from a seat or climbing steps and stairs. If your shoulders or hands are affected, you may find that reaching into cabinets, plugging in electrical appliances, or turning on faucets may be a problem.

Getting into and around your home

A grab rail beside the front or back door will help you manage the steps into your home. You may need a ramp—a gradient of one in 12 is recommended if you are a wheelchair user. For the stairs, an extra banister rail may be all you need to steady yourself. There are many types of stair lifts on the market for those who need more help and a through-floor elevator will benefit wheelchair users.

If you use a wheelchair or walker indoors, you will need a little more space to allow you to turn in a room and to move from one room to another. Removing an internal wall can improve your access and mobility in the home.

Help with rising

People with arthritis find that a chair designed with a high seat and back as well as arm rests is relaxing to sit in. It is also easier to get up from such a chair than from a low three-piece sofa. You can raise the seat of your chair by placing a deep cushion on it or by fitting a specially made chair raise unit under it. A powered riser-recliner chair with an elevating leg rest is ideal.

Your toilet may be raised by building a base under it or by fitting it with a raised toilet seat. These come with or without rails. Alternatively, a grab rail fitted to the wall may help you rise from the toilet. If arthritis affects your arms and hands, toilets can be equipped with a washing and drying facility.

Beds can be raised on blocks to help you stand up when you get up. A rail fitted to the bed can help you sit up from a prone position. For even more assistance, try using a powered pillow or mattress lifter.

Taking a shower is easier than getting out of a bath and a walk-in shower is easiest to access. A grab rail on the wall or a seat can be helpful in a shower or a bath. If you prefer to soak in a warm bath and need more help to get out, try a power-rise bath seat, with or without a reclining back rest.

Ergonomic design

A good ergonomic design in the home may involve altering the height of work surfaces and cabinets, raising or lowering appliances and electric outlets

Wearing a splint can support and protect unstable and painful joints in your body.

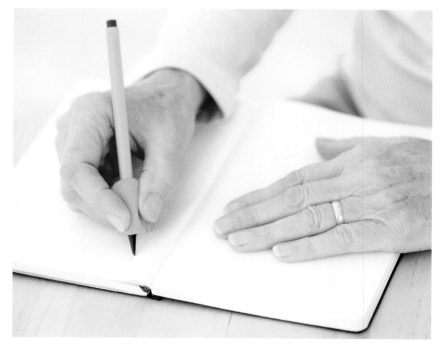

PEN GRIP
Writing is easier with a pen grip because you don't have to press hard and you experience less pain and fatigue.

to enable you to gain access, and ensuring that controls and handles are easy to grip. The sink, stove, and work surface of your kitchen's "working triangle" should be close together, at the same height, and without obstruction.

Assistive devices

Using assistive devices or gadgets will help you cope with the difficulties arthritis causes. They may be familiar products that you can find in any supply store or else specifically designed to help overcome a particular disability.

For example, electric can openers are widely available and are less effort than opening with a manual gadget. However, you will need to find a store specializing in such equipment to purchase a sock aid (which helps you put socks on when you cannot reach your feet).

You may be able to borrow some of the larger items from arthritic aid groups.

Personal care
Pain and stiffness in shoulders, back, and hips can make it hard to reach down to put on shoes and socks, or to reach up to brush hair, shave, or put on shirts.

Various long-handled gadgets will help with most problems—for example, long-handled shoehorn, sponge, hair brush, and "helping

hand." A stick with a hook at one end and a rubber thimble at the other can help hook pants over your feet or push shirts off your shoulders. It is best to choose clothing with few fastenings if your grip is weak.

A button hook can be helpful and tying a loop on a zipper gives a better grip. Choose chunky grips or use an electric toothbrush or razor. Try moist toilet tissue if using the ordinary kind is difficult.

General household needs
A wide range of gadgets are available to help you with many of your general household needs:
● Jar, bottle, and can openers.
● Wide-handled peelers, chunky cutlery, and ergonomic knives with upright handles.
● Lever gadgets for faucets, door handles, keys, and plugs.
● Long-handled dustpan and brush.
● Teapot tippers.
● Self-opening scissors.

LONG-HANDLED DUSTPAN AND BRUSH

Long handles so you can stand upright.

Dust pan swivels so you don't need to bend over.

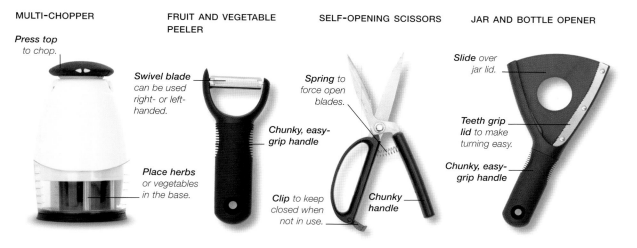

MULTI-CHOPPER

Press top to chop.

FRUIT AND VEGETABLE PEELER

Swivel blade can be used right- or left-handed.

Place herbs or vegetables in the base.

SELF-OPENING SCISSORS

Spring to force open blades.

Chunky, easy-grip handle

Clip to keep closed when not in use.

Chunky handle

JAR AND BOTTLE OPENER

Slide over jar lid.

Teeth grip lid to make turning easy.

Chunky, easy-grip handle

• Contour grips to turn knobs and dials.
• Book rests and pen grips.
• Wrist rests, adapted keyboards, and mouse control for computers.

Family life and looking after children

Raising a family can be the most rewarding and productive time in life. Families make many demands of us, however, both physically and emotionally. Pain, fatigue, and disability caused by arthritis can combine to interfere with your role as an active parent.

A survey of grandparents and parents with arthritis revealed that the most common childcare problems were lifting a baby or child from the floor or from a crib, getting children to help with household chores, and having enough energy to keep up with children (see right).

Arthritis has an impact on every aspect of family life; how family members feel about and relate to each other, how roles and responsibilities are taken on, and how decisions are made.

If you are a parent with arthritis, you may feel guilty about not being able to do all the things you think you should. It may not be possible to walk your children to school, play football with them, or go out in the evening with your partner because you feel too tired.

At the same time, the pain and inflammation you feel may make you more irritable and you may take it out on those nearest you, or push them away when they offer help or comfort.

Family members who are eager to help you can unintentionally contribute to your feelings of helplessness, frustration, and dependence. This is especially true when they jump in too quickly and immediately take over all the

KITCHEN TOOLS
A range of kitchen tools make many food preparation tasks easier and less painful.

PRACTICAL TIPS

LOOKING AFTER BABIES AND CHILDREN

• Make sure you can use baby equipment safely and manage the fastenings.

• Change diapers where you don't need to stoop.

• When bathing a baby use a sculpted foam cushion and nonslip mat. On "bad" days, just use a mat and sponge.

• Manage your energy so you have enough for play.

• Get children to help you by making household tasks into a game.

• Read books together—it allows you to rest.

• Encourage children to climb gently onto your knee.

jobs that you find difficult or painful. You will need to negotiate the amount of help you want to keep some of your independence.

Your family can be a major source of emotional and practical support and it is very important to communicate honestly with them. Just as you may have had difficulty accepting that you have arthritis, your family may find it difficult to come to terms with, too. Explain to them about arthritis and how you feel, and encourage them to ask questions. This will help them see past the problems to the real you and help them come to terms with the limitations imposed by your condition.

Personal relationships

Arthritis does not just affect you in isolation—it can potentially affect everyone who comes into contact with you. Good communication is the key in maintaining all your relationships, whether platonic or sexual. For people with arthritis this is equally, if not more, vital.

Communication takes effort so that when you are in pain or feeling tired you may find you don't have the energy. Be honest about how you feel—those closest to you need to know. Sometimes it is hard to explain your arthritis, so give an information leaflet to your family and work colleagues. The

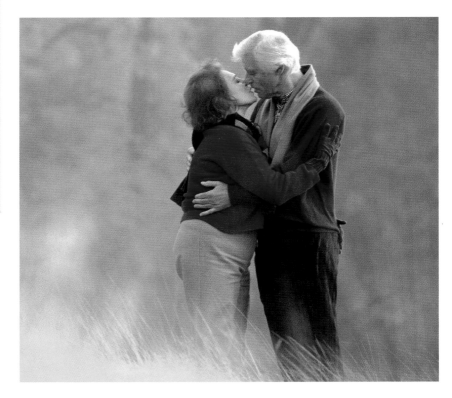

A LOVING RELATIONSHIP
People with arthritis can expect to share in the joy and pleasure of a loving relationship.

differences between the types of arthritis are not understood very well. Ask your physician or rheumatologist (see useful addresses, p.215) for a leaflet.

Sexuality and sexual relationships

Sexuality is an important part of who we are. We express this in different ways: in the way we dress, present ourselves, and communicate—both verbally and nonverbally. Many people express themselves within a sexual relationship. Arthritis can have a negative impact on your sexuality and sexual relationships, so it is important that you address issues as they arise (see Sexual relationships, opposite).

Traveling and moving around

Pain and fatigue can restrict your independence and reduce the frequency and length of time you can spend traveling. The following advice can help you improve your ability to get around:

■ **COMFORTABLE FOOTWEAR** Make sure your footwear gives you the maximum amount of comfort. Sneakers or thick-soled shoes are best. It can be difficult to find footwear that looks good and is comfortable. Ask your podiatrist, health professional, or a good shoe store for advice.

■ **WALKING AIDS** Various types of walking aids are available. There are special handles, which can reduce the stress on hand and upper limb joints that are affected by arthritis. It is best to get advice from a physical therapist who will be able to tell you what walking aids are most suitable for you.

■ **WHEELCHAIRS AND SCOOTERS** Wheelchairs and scooters are often seen as a last resort and this perception is understandable. They can, however, provide valuable independence and increased opportunity to travel and socialize.

Standard manual wheelchairs may be provided by arthritis aid societies but if you want nonstandard models then you may need to buy them yourself. Try out a variety of models before you make your choice, and discuss your needs with your occupational and physical therapists.

■ **DRIVING** Driving can be a real challenge, depending on the type of car you have, how far you are traveling, and the severity of your arthritis.

If you believe that arthritis may be affecting your ability to drive, ask your physician to refer you to a rehabilitation center or a specialist, or see Useful Addresses, p.215. These people can determine whether or not you drive safely, if there are any special devices that might facilitate your driving, and they may offer training in using

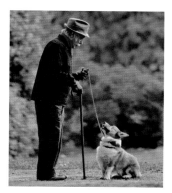

WALKING AIDS
Various sturdy walking aids can help provide support, stability, and balance.

Your family can be a major source of emotional and practical support.

these devices as well as improving your driving skills.

If you have difficulty traveling by car, there are a number of things you can do to make the trip easier. For instance, it may help to take your analgesics and/or anti-inflammatory drugs at a particular time before the trip starts so that they are working effectively when you most need them. However, make sure that your medications don't make you sleepy; otherwise, you could be arrested for driving under the influence.

■ **TRAINS, BOATS, AND PLANES** These forms of transportation can be more relaxing and less stressful than driving a car, especially on long trips. Train stations, ferry terminals, and airports should be accessible under the Americans with Disabilities Act (1990). It is always worth calling your travel agent to tell him or her what assistance you are likely to need so that it can be arranged.

Occupational therapists

People with arthritis can turn to an occupational therapist for help in achieving their personal, work, domestic, educational, or leisure goals. Occupational therapists can help you improve your ability to perform routine tasks, make lifestyle changes, and prevent or reduce your chances of losing roles and abilities in the future.

Q&A

I have great difficulty parking my car near the stores—what assistance can I get?

Under the ADA Accessibiliy Guidelines for Buildings and Facilities, parking lots must have some parking spaces that are close to the entrance. To use one of these spaces, you must obtain a Disabled Parking placard from your local Department of Motor Vehicles.

A rheumatologist can refer you to a rheumatology occupational therapist who specializes in solving the problems caused by arthritis. Either on your own or through a referral from your health professional, you can contact the occupational therapists at the local hospital for larger pieces of equipment or home adaptations.

How occupational therapists can help

Occupational therapists can help in a number of ways, usually when you are in hospital or when you are at home. Some may see you at a school or university, or at work. Occupational therapists can advise you on all the sections in this chapter—from household chores, home modifications, and assistive devices, to work, travel, asking for help, family life, and childcare.

Usually, occupational therapists will assess and treat you on a one-to-one basis. However, they may invite you to attend group sessions. Occupational therapists can help by:

● Discussing practical problems and showing you how you can overcome them. These could include problems at home, work, school, and further education or with your leisure pursuits.

● Teaching you how to look after your joints. It is important that you understand as much as possible how your arthritis affects your joints and what you can do in your day-to-day activities to help you get the most out them. This includes teaching you how to minimize the strain you put on your joints.

● Teaching you physical or psychological techniques to manage your pain and fatigue.

● Helping you return to former activities or teaching new activities to help you achieve your goals.

● Making splints to rest or support painful or damaged joints.

Asking for help

Ask for what you need—it will improve your chances of getting it. When you have arthritis, you don't have to battle alone. Acknowledge your limitations and accept help without feeling guilty. Having someone do the jobs that hurt or tire you will save you energy and reduce frustration. Friends may be able to help with shopping, children with household chores,

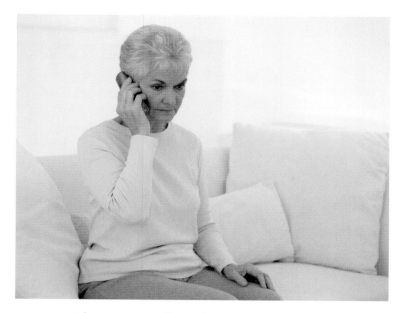

partners with getting you dressed. You will be better company for those around you! Plan ahead, figure out what you need and who your helpers are (see also p.132).

Learn as much as you can about your arthritis and how it can be managed. Get to know the health professionals who can help and call them when you need to. Many rheumatology departments have telephone helplines.

Community services can advise you on home adaptations or financial support. They may be able to organize help for you with your shopping or personal care.

Look for a self-management program in your area for people who have long-term medical conditions. This gives people the opportunity to support each other and swap tips. Ask your physician or rheumatologist for details.

HELPLINES
Various support services and rheumatology departments have set up helplines that you can contact for advice.

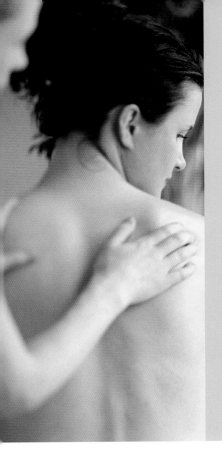

Coping with pain

People with arthritis usually have mild to moderate pain, stiffness, and inflammation in their joints. From time to time, these symptoms flare up and make the arthritis feel much worse. Flare-ups may be attributable to excessive use of the joints but are often bewilderingly inexplicable and unpredictable, causing a great deal of anxiety. When healthcare professionals are not available to treat your flare-ups, you can turn to some simple, safe, and effective means for coping with your pain and managing your arthritis. These remedies can also reduce inflammation and stiffness and improve your quality of life.

Reducing pain helps you regain control of your independence and manage your arthritis better.

What causes pain?

Pain is the response of the nervous system when an injury or disease damages the tissues of the body. It is often thought of as a simple alarm system that stimulates the body to take protective action to avoid additional damage. However, as anyone who regularly feels pain will tell you, there are types of persistent (chronic) pain that defy all reason and seem to serve no purpose whatsoever.

The type of pain depends on the person who is experiencing it as well as on its cause. Different people will feel pain in different ways. Some have a low threshold and feel low levels of pain more acutely than others, who seem able to withstand intense pain without complaint. Personality and mood can also determine the way you feel pain—stress, fear, and anxiety can all make pain feel worse.

The pain gate

How the pain response mechanism actually works is something of a mystery. One explanation, called the pain gate theory, can help you understand the effects of pain and its management.

According to the theory, there is a pain gate through which nervous impulses carrying the message of pain must pass. Normally the gate is closed but when a pain hurts so much—for example, in a flare-up that irritates the nerves in the skin, joints, and muscles—the nervous impulses pass through the gate and reach the brain, where the pain is registered and interpreted.

Various remedies have the effect of shutting—or at least partly blocking—the pain gate. On the other hand, stress and anxiety can open the gate or make it easier for the nerve impulses to pass through.

Relieving pain

The body has its own way of relieving pain, at least for short periods. The brain and spinal cord produce endorphins and encephalins that belong to the same chemical family as morphine and have a similar sedative effect.

Treating pain

Flare-ups affect many people with chronic and fluctuating conditions, particularly rheumatoid arthrits but also osteoarthritis. They can last for weeks or months before they subside and better days return.

There are many different ways of treating pain when it flares up. Doctors prescribe drugs and occupational therapists, physical therapists, nurses, and podiatrists (who treat feet) use various kinds of interventions.

However, it is a good idea to discover ways of coping with your own unique pain. Then, when your symptoms of pain, swelling, and inflammation flare up, you are not as reliant on your physician or healthcare professional because you have your own ways of managing your symptoms.

Ways to reduce pain

Reducing pain helps you regain control of your independence and manage your arthritis better. There are a number of ways you can choose to reduce your pain, such as massage, applying heat or cold, and breathing and relaxation exercises. You may also find that they make your pain-reliving medication work better.

Some remedies work by releasing naturally occurring endorphins while others reduce your muscle tension, which helps decrease pain and improves the blood supply to muscles to enable freer movement.

Massage

Massage relieves muscle tension, improves circulation, and disperses the fluid in swollen joints and muscles. It is a natural reaction to pain. Rubbing shuts the pain gate by stimulating the nerves in the skin, muscles, and joints, thereby blocking pain signals.

PRACTICAL TIPS

MANAGING FLARE-UPS

● Rest, but not in bed. Avoid or reduce activities that aggravate your pain—for example, prolonged standing or walking—for a couple of days until the pain subsides.

● Use heat or cold (or whatever you find eases your pain) several times each day (see p.148).

● If you feel anxious and tense, practice deep breathing and relaxation techniques (see p.150) to help you calm down.

● Resume exercising gently once the pain starts to settle. If you do not move, your joints will stiffen up and your muscles will weaken and tire quickly.

● Reestablish your action plan (see p.73) and increase your activity levels gradually.

PRACTICAL TIPS

APPLYING HEAT OR COLD

● Lie down in a comfortable position and relax before applying either heat or cold treatment.

● To apply heat, place a heat pack or a hot-water bottle wrapped in a towel on the painful, inflamed joint for 10–15 minutes.

● To apply cold, place a cool pack or a bag of frozen peas wrapped in a towel on the painful, inflamed joint for 10–15 minutes.

● Remove the pack (either hot or cold) and gently move your joint. The combination of movement and rest is very important for pain relief.

● Replace the heat pack on the joint for another 5–10 minutes.

The physical contact in massage has been shown to be profoundly comforting, probably by releasing endorphins and encephalins, which reduce heart and breathing rates. Some of the pain relief from by moisturizers, lotions, oils, gels, and creams is probably due to the massage needed to apply them.

Gently massaging painful joints or muscles for 5–10 minutes is a very effective, safe, and pleasurable way to relieve pain.

Heat and cold

People with arthritis often apply heat and cold to a joint to control the pain of their flare-ups (see p.149). Hot and cold sensations increase the nerve impulses that block pain signals and shut the pain gate. In addition, heat is particularly good at relaxing tense muscles. Both heat and cold improve your blood supply, reduce swelling, and enable you to move more freely,

Warmth created by commercially available heat packs, a hot-water bottle wrapped in a towel, taking a hot bath, and wearing thermal clothing or bandages can reduce pain considerably.

Cooling can be produced with commercially available cool packs, coolant sprays, or a bag of frozen peas wrapped in a towel.

For most people, warming or cooling a joint is a safe technique. However, people who have circulatory problems should consult their physician, physical therapist, or nurse. Make sure you don't burn your skin with a heat pack or hot-water bottle. Whatever method you use, avoid becoming uncomfortably hot or cold.

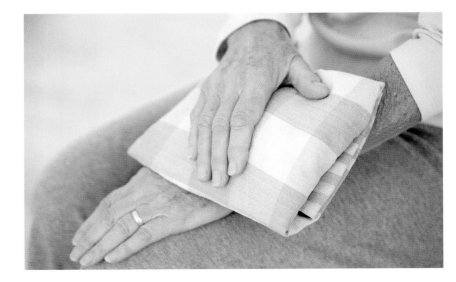

FROZEN PEAS
The cool temperature of a bag of frozen peas can relieve pain, improve the supply of blood, and reduce swelling.

Water therapy

For thousands of years, people have used water therapy to treat arthritic conditions. Water therapy relieves pain by using the warmth and buoyancy of water to relax muscles and reduce the weight-bearing load and stress on your legs and trunk.

Spa therapy

This residential treatment involves bathing in naturally heated water (often rich in minerals), hot mud packs, respite care, and gentle movement. Its effectiveness lies, at least in part, in the absence of domestic pressures, the relaxing environment, and a holistic health approach. However, it is expensive and has limited availability.

Hydrotherapy

This form of spa therapy uses the buoyancy, assistance, and resistance properties of warm water to help you exercise more effectively. It is cheaper than spa therapy but still requires dedicated facilities and therapists. Many medical insurance plans cover this therapy.

Aquatherapy

A growing number of community pools run aquatherapy classes. They provide many people with the opportunity to participate in controlled water-based exercise classes, supervised by experienced therapists at moderate cost.

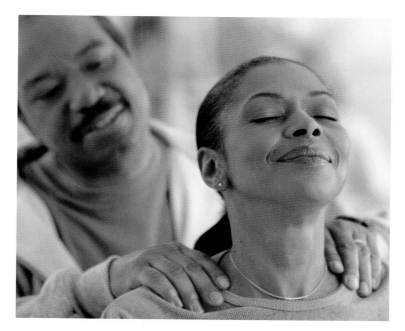

Aquatherapy offers most of the benefits of hydrotherapy to many more people for longer. If you cannot find an aquatherapy class, exercise gently in your local swimming pool to keep your stiff and painful joints moving.

THE POWER OF TOUCH
Massage brings relaxation and calm to tense muscles and painful joints, thereby illustrating the healing power of touch.

Electrical stimulation

Transcutaneous electrical neuromuscular stimulation (TENS) is a self-administered, noninvasive form of pain control that many people have found helpful. This treatment may work both by shutting the pain gate and by stimulating the release of endorphins and encephalins, which help relieve your pain, relax your tense muscles, and slow your breathing.

Water therapy relieves pain by using the warmth and buoyancy of water to relax muscles and reduce the weight-bearing load and stress on your legs and trunk.

Although physical therapists use several different pieces of electrical equipment to reduce pain, the best scientific evidence supports TENS as being the most effective of these.

TENS machines are readily available at a reasonable cost and for home use. Consult your physician before you start using a TENS machine and ask a physical therapist to show you how to use it.

A TENS machine is a safe way of relieving pain. It delivers small electrical pulses that pass through electrodes taped to the skin where you are feeling pain. You can use it for up to 24 hours, whether you are sitting, standing, or gently moving around.

Don't use a TENS machine if you are pregnant, or if you have a pacemaker or heart condition. Never place the electrodes near the carotid artery in your neck.

Relaxation and breathing

When you are in pain you start to think the worst of everything. You become stressed, exacerbating your negative thoughts (see p.154) and increasing your feeling of being helplessly controlled by pain. You need to break this vicious circle in order to regain control over your life as well as your symptoms.

The first step that you need to take is to recognize the signs of increased stress, tension, and anxiety. These include shallow breathing, feeling uptight, and being nervous.

Notice how situations that make you stressed and anxious increase the muscle tension in your neck, shoulders, back, and legs. Notice, too, how these feelings are associated with pain. Therefore, try to avoid such situations and learn some techniques that will help you manage your condition and relax, feel happier, and sleep better.

Two quick exercises

Many relaxation techniques can help reduce tension and anxiety. The most common involve deep breathing and exercises that contract and relax your muscles in a progressive way.

There are two quick exercises that you can practice almost any time, any place, anywhere (see left and opposite). Practice them when you are not stressed so that you can become more confident in your ability.

At first you may be sceptical that such simple relaxation techniques will help you control your pain, but try them and see. If they don't work, at least you can say you have tried and will have lost little. On the other hand, if these techniques do work, you will gain a great deal.

PRACTICAL TIPS

DEEP BREATHING

● Sit or stand up straight without forcefully breathing. Gently breath in, allowing your chest to expand fully.

● Relax your shoulders.

● Place a hand on your abdomen just below your ribcage.

● Take a slow, deep breath in through your nose—feel your hand and stomach rising up.

● When your lungs are fully expanded, slowly breath out through your mouth—feel your abdomen and hand gently sink.

● Repeat this for 4 or 5 deep breaths, then rest and breath in a normal relaxed way for a couple of minutes. If necessary, repeat the exercise for 5–10 minutes.

Alternating activity with rest

Physical activity is unquestionably good for controlling arthritic pain, but so, too, are rest and relaxation. Try to avoid getting tired because it leads to muscle weakness, which increases the risk of further pain and joint damage.

Most people begin to experience pain after doing an activity for a relatively short time but they continue with the task until it is completed or pain becomes so bad that they are forced to rest.

Periods of rest

A better solution is to limit the time you spend doing the activity by interspersing it with periods of rest. You can then continue your normal activities within bearable limits of pain and discomfort.

First identify the activities that cause you pain and think about the way you are doing them. Find out how long each activity takes to start making you feel tired or have some mild discomfort, then take a short rest. For example, if after 20 minutes of gardening you feel discomfort, rest for 5–10 minutes, then return to the task. Take another break if pain starts to increase again or finish the task another time.

If you record your activity–rest times you will find that the activity time increases before you need to rest, and the activity becomes much easier with much less pain.

PRACTICAL TIPS

MUSCLE RELAXATION

● Stop whatever activity you are doing. Stand, sit, or (preferably) lie down somewhere quiet.

● Take a few deep breaths. If you're anxious your breathing will be quick and shallow, which will make you uptight.

● Close your eyes and imagine a relaxing scene, such as sitting on a quiet beach on a sunny day.

● Starting from your shoulders, tighten your muscles, hold them tight for 5 seconds, then relax.

● Feel the tension release from your muscles and joints. They will feel looser and make you feel lighter. Work through each muscle group, from the top of your body to your toes.

● Hold onto that feeling of relaxation for 30 seconds before returning to the activity you were doing.

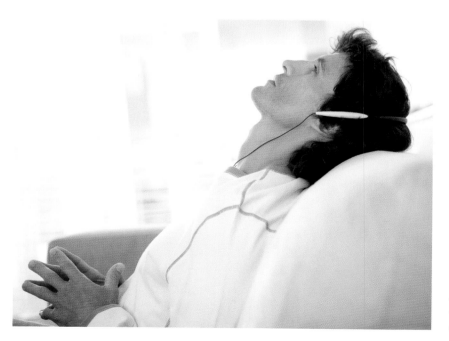

RELAXATION
One of the best ways to cope with your pain is relaxation—it relieves tense muscles, calms you down, and gives you back control.

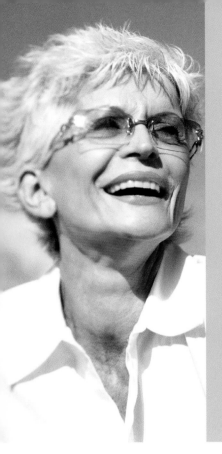

Coping with stress

Living with the ups and downs of arthritis can disturb your emotional state so that you feel frustration, anger, guilt, sadness, loss, fear, anxiety, or hurt. At times it can be an emotional roller-coaster, especially when you are diagnosed or during periods of yet more pain, fatigue, or uncertainty about your treatment or the future. Emotional changes can increase your levels of stress while your negative thoughts and beliefs can fuel the vicious cycle of pain, fatigue, and stress. Psychological ways of managing stress can break this cycle, reducing your pain and fatigue, and helping to make you happier.

Whatever the situation, you can choose how you wish to react to it because you have a measure of free will.

What is stress?

Stress is a part of life. You can feel it in the painful, anxious, exciting, depressing, irritating, dangerous, or frightening experiences that affect us all every single day.

Stress is also the way your body and mind respond to each of these stressors—chemically in the way your nerves work, physically in the way your body responds, and psychologically in the way your mind reacts (see opposite).

Sources of stress can be found in changes to your lifestyle (such as work, family, finances, home, and friends), imagined changes (such as fears about the future and about your inability to do things), and everyday hassles (such as traffic jams, lines, noise, problems at work, and bad news on TV). The symptoms and effects of arthritis are also a source of stress. Stress itself also increases the symptoms of arthritis.

When faced with a potential stressor you wonder if you can cope. If you believe you can, your stress response is less likely to be activated. If you believe you can't, or are faced with too many hassles, worries, and physical problems, you are more likely to be stressed and emotionally upset.

Changing your responses to stress

You need to release stress before it builds up and starts to dominate your life. Many methods can help relieve stress, including exercise, movement therapies, relaxation, breathing techniques, meditation.

The mind is also a powerful tool in dealing with stress. One of the advantages of using psychological approaches to stress is that you can be in control of what happens inside your own mind. Whatever the situation, you can choose how you wish to react to it because you have a measure of free will. Our attitudes, thoughts, and beliefs shape our responses to stress—not events, past or present. Changing the way you think takes work and mental effort, especially if you have been under stress for a long time. However, with perseverance the rewards are a happier outlook in life and better health.

The ABC method

Cognitive therapists and life coaches, who can help us unravel and understand the mental knots and confused thinking that affects us all, have developed very

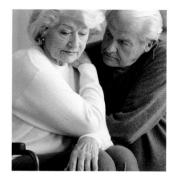

TALKING HELPS
The stress of some situations and thoughts that can be eased simply by talking them through with a person who cares for you.

THE BODY'S REACTION TO STRESS

When you are stressed, a range of chemical, physical, and psychological changes occur within you. Many of the physical and psychological changes are like the symptoms you may experience as you cope with the pain and inflammation of arthritis. It is important to recognize stress and realize that it can contribute to some of your pain, fatigue, muscle tension, and sleep problems. Stress management techniques can reduce these symptoms and help you to cope with your arthritis.

CHEMICAL CHANGES

- The body produces higher levels of three hormones—epinephrine, norepinephrine, and cortisol. These increase heart rate, blood pressure, respiration, and metabolism, and lead to the release of chemicals that control the functions of the body's systems.

- The brain produces less of the hormone serotonin, thereby causing sleep disturbance.

PHYSICAL CHANGES

- Breathing becomes faster and shallower

- Tense muscles

- Heart rate quickens

- Skin may be clammy

If stress levels stay high:
- Increased fatigue, aches, and pains

- Stomach and bowel disturbances

- Headaches

- Raised blood pressure

- Loss of appetite

PSYCHOLOGICAL CHANGES

- Increased worrying or irritability

- Increased depression

- Images of losing control and being helpless

- Poorer concentration and memory

- Poorer self-image, less self-belief

- Increased automatic negative thoughts

- Restlessness, accident proneness, poorer time management, lower productivity.

What you want to develop is a logical, rational approach to dispute your thoughts.

effective strategies for coping with stress. One of these, the ABC method, may help you understand how you respond to a stressful event and how you can change your response. A is the Activating event, B represents the Beliefs and thoughts that are triggered in your mind, and C summarizes the Consequences—the emotional, physical, or behavioral changes.

When some event happens that triggers a stress response inside you, particularly when you have been under a lot of stress, there may be negative consequences. For instance, you get emotionally upset and your pain and fatigue get worse. This activating event seems to lead to the consequences, but is this really true? Perhaps the event is the last straw and that other, more deep-seated problems are causing the consequences.

Identify negative thoughts

The first step to changing the nature of your stress response is to identify the beliefs and thoughts that run through your mind.

As we become progressively stressed, we get more emotionally upset and are likely to think more and more automatic negative thoughts (ANTs). These are called automatic because the negative thoughts just pop into our minds involuntarily and, at the time, are very believable.

The higher your stress levels, the more you believe these ANTs are true. They run through your mind and become difficult to shift. They trigger more negative thoughts and increase your stress response still further. ANTs can become a habit, like thinking traps you fall into time and again.

However, once you start to identify your ANTs, you can start changing them. Be honest with yourself about the thinking traps you can fall into—for example:
- All or nothing thinking—you see things in extremes.
- Mind reading—you know what others are thinking without first hearing what they have to say.
- Personalization—you blame yourself for events that are not your responsibility.
- Emotional reasoning—you feel something strongly therefore it must be true.
- Labeling—you often attach a negative label to an event.

TRAFFIC JAMS
One of the most irritating sources of stress is a traffic jam—it very rarely fails to trigger a negative response that leaves us feeling tense and anxious.

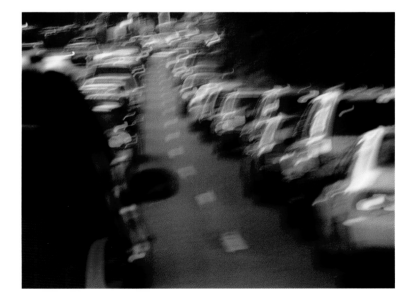

USING A THOUGHT AND SYMPTOM DIARY (THE ABCDE METHOD)

Keep a diary that records the dates and activating events that trigger stress. Fill it in as soon as you can while the event is fresh in your mind. Record your thoughts, beliefs, emotions, and the consequences. Then compose your disputing thoughts that put a positive spin on the event and the effective actions to take next time. In this example, a woman with rheumatoid arthritis feels stress because her two boys won't put on their coats for school and end up rushing to catch the bus.

BELIEFS/THOUGHTS	CONSEQUENCES	DISPUTING THOUGHTS	EFFECTIVE ACTIONS
• "I'll never get them to school on time." • "I'm such an awful mother!" • "I can never cope with these kids, I'm useless!" • "Every morning is one long struggle!"	• Feel frustrated, hassled. Tense muscles. Tired. • Shallow breathing, heart racing, feel stressed. • Later in day, pain and fatigue worse. Headache. Worrying. • Difficult managing so many jobs.	• "Most of the time we manage to get to the bus on time." • "Being a bit late sometimes is OK." • "I can cope with the kids. In fact, most of the time I do cope."	• Take deep breaths. • Give them a kiss—the boys always want to get away then! • Get lunch ready the night before to avoid rushing in the morning. • Talk to the boys about why I need them to help.

• Discounting the positive—you see things negatively and push aside any positive experiences or personal qualities that you have.
• Fortune-telling—you believe you have the power to predict the future accurately.
• Musts and shoulds—you steadfastly abide by internal rules that cannot be broken.

Develop an effective outlook

The next step in changing the way you think is to build on your ABC. Add a D and an E by Disputing your negative thoughts and beliefs, then develop an Effective outlook.

In hindsight, we look back at negative thoughts and rationally think "Of course I see now that isn't true." What you want to develop is a logical, rational approach to dispute your thoughts and avoid the consequences at the time of the stressful event, to keep from sliding into emotional distress. Such an approach will help train your mind to have a more positive, flexible, resilient, and effective outlook, so that you are better able to cope with stress-triggering events in the future.

Keep a thought and symptom diary (see above) to help you focus on the various aspects of the ABCDE model and to complete the process of changing the way you think. Once you have identified your negative thoughts, start disputing them. Try the following:
• What is the evidence for the thoughts you are thinking?
• Are you applying double standards to yourself?

MEDITATION
One of the best ways to quiet your mind and relax the body is to practice meditation every day.

PRACTICAL TIPS

KEEPING A JOURNAL

Here are some ideas to put in your journal:

● A thought and symptom diary (see p.155) to help you see the link between thoughts, feelings, stress and worsening arthritis symptoms. Keep track of your disputing thoughts and other coping ideas.

● Problem-solving for practical solutions.

● Records of exercises and activities.

● Effectiveness of drugs, complementary therapies, and diet.

● Keep a record of how well you sleep and how often you wake at night.

● Goal-setting (see p.73).

● Think in shades of gray instead of in all or nothing terms. Give different aspects of an event a score on a scale of 0–100.
● Why are you calling yourself names for failing at something?
● Change the musts and shoulds and ease up on yourself.
● List the pros and cons of your negative thought, feeling, or behavior. This is good for developing a rational perspective.
● Develop positive statements and find inspirational sayings to write on cards (keep them in your pocket, bag, or on the fridge door to remind you) or in a journal. Read these to affirm to yourself your abilities and positive actions.
● Use other coping strategies that will help, such as deep breathing techniques (see p.150), relaxation training (see pp.150–151), and the planning ahead principles in joint protection (see p.176).

Mind–body exercises

Meditation, deep breathing (see p.150), and visualization (see p.157) are effective exercises that reduce stress. They can help restore a more balanced outlook on life, reduce tension, and lower blood pressure. Practice them regularly—preferably, every day.

Meditation

This mind–body technique is an excellent way to create a relaxed state of awareness. Meditation helps you to develop calmness, improve your concentration, and relieve pain, stress, and depression. Try the following sequence:

Find the right time, such as the morning or before bed. You will develop skills more quickly if you practice regularly. Start for just 5 or 10 minutes, a few times a week.

Find the right place—a quiet special place where there are no interruptions and where the room is warm. Personalize it with a meditation object you like—for example, a candle, a favorite stone, a remarkable pine cone, a beautiful flower, or an appealing painting. Burn incense and play soothing music if you wish.

Sit down or lie comfortably. Support your head and keep your back straight so you can breathe freely and deeply. Wearing loose clothes will help, too.

Quiet your body with deep breathing. Focus on your special meditation object (either in reality or in your mind) as your focal point. Don't try too hard. Let your feelings and thoughts drift in and out of your consciousness without becoming involved in them.

Gradually imagine the feelings and thoughts are like ripples in a pond, moving away from you.

Stay focused on your breathing. If you become distracted, don't worry—just bring your attention back to your focal point. Whatever you feel—peaceful, bored, or tense—is normal. It takes time to develop inner stillness. As you practice regularly, so you will find that it becomes easier.

When you feel calmer, center your mind on the word "peace". Meditate on this word and let it fill both your mind and body.

After a few minutes, release the word "peace" so that only the essence of peace remains within you. Notice how relaxed you feel. Breathe deeply and gradually focus your mind back to the room.

Give yourself time to persevere with meditation. Before long it will grow more and more effective.

VISUALIZATION

This mind–body exercise can be a powerful way of relaxing. It is also called guided imagery because you guide yourself through a relaxing scene and let your troubles ebb away.

A number of visualization CDs are available—try to find one you like, then sit or lie comfortably with your arms and legs relaxed.

Alternatively, you could devise your own sequence and either record and listen to it, or learn it and repeat it to yourself. The following excerpt from a sequence may inspire you:

"Breathe deeply through your nose and exhale slowly through your mouth. Again, take a deep breath in slowly...and slowly exhale...feel your tension melt away...your body feels heavy and warm...listen to your heart beat.

"Imagine you are on a warm beach, by a quiet calm sea...as the water gently laps inhale and exhale...one after the other your negative emotions ebb away...like the waves on the sand...worries... frustration...pain...sadness...ebb away. You're content...at peace... relaxed...happier...lighter..."

When you're ready, end the exercise by wiggling your fingers and toes, and return to the every day feeling refreshed.

RELAXING SCENE
A good focus for visualization is a gentle scene where waves break rhythmically on a sandy shore.

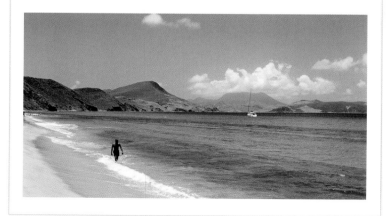

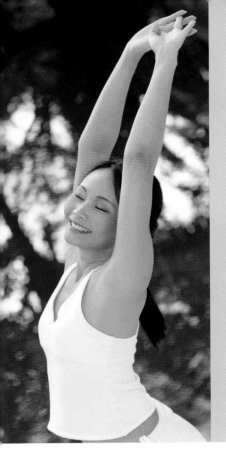

Maintaining your mobility

Arthritis can seriously limit your ability to do things and so you may be tempted, even encouraged, to rest and become less active. Although this is understandable, it would be a mistake because you would start to lose your mobility and your flexibility. All the activities you enjoy, such as walking, dancing, swimming, or cycling, become increasingly hard to do. The exercises that follow will help you maintain and improve your mobility so that you can manage your arthritis more effectively.

Follow the exercise routine

Before you start, read the "Ten Exercise Rules" (see opposite). The first rule is the most important: whatever exercise you do, make sure you are both stable and safe. Always have something solid to grab—but make sure that it will support you.

In the exercises on the following pages, the head turns, head rolls, sit-to-stands, step-ups, and squats can make you feel dizzy, so be very careful. If possible, do them with someone beside you. You can either do every exercise as part of a daily plan or focus on individual exercises according to your needs.

Start with low-impact exercises that do not involve your bearing any weight. These are the ones in which you sit or lie on the floor or on a bed. Then build up to doing the weight-bearing exercises and functional activities, such as walking (see p.157).

Two groups of exercises

The exercises in this chapter can be classified into two groups. The first group are the flexibility exercises, which use minimal resistance to increase or maintain the range of movement of your

Q&A

How can I tell if I have done too much exercise?

It is normal that doing a new or unusual activity will make your joints and muscles ache a little. However, if the pain and discomfort continues to increase, lasts for more than two days, is accompanied by swelling of the joint, or wakes you at night you have probably overdone things. Rest for a few days to allow everything to settle down, then resume your exercising and build up slowly.

joints. The second group of exercises use a resistance (such as an elastic band or your body weight) to increase strength.

In both these types of exercises, try to "nudge the boundaries" of your capabilities, challenging yourself to gently, gradually move a little farther or work a little harder. Once you have reached a level you are content with, continue that level of exercise to maintain the progress you have achieved. If you continually do less and less you will slip back and lose mobility.

Performing the exercises well, with controlled movement, is as important as repeating the exercise more often or for longer. In addition, try to hold the position at the end of a range-of-movement exercise, such as the shoulder rotation, so that you feel a gentle stretch. Keep your breathing relaxed as you do this because

it increases the effectiveness of the stretch and maximizes your effort. Being too forceful and enthusiastic or "aggressive" can increase pain and discomfort.

Adapt the guidelines

In the exercises that follow, the instructions suggest how long you could hold a particular movement and how many repetitions of an exercise you can do—but these are just guidelines. Some people may be able to do more right from the beginning, others less.

Adapt the guidelines to suit you, but be careful if you are not used to exercising: what seems like a simple and easy task can cause discomfort and pain, which may lead to anxiety that you caused damage by doing too much. Err on the side of caution—start gently and increase gradually.

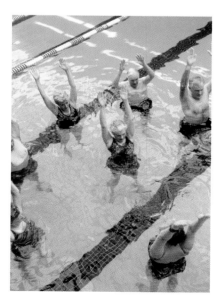

WATER EXERCISE
Warm-water swimming pools are good places to exercise many of your joints and improve their mobility and flexibility.

PRACTICAL TIPS

TEN EXERCISE RULES

● When doing an exercise always make sure you're stable and safe. For example, if you stand, have something near to hold.

● Start each new exercise gently and cautiously.

● Increase the amount or kind of exercise gradually over days and weeks.

● Work hard but don't cause prolonged pain or discomfort.

● Rest on days when your joints are painful. When the pain subsides, resume exercising gently.

● Perform the exercises using well-controlled movement—quality is as important as quantity.

● Set yourself realistic goals.

● Write an action plan and tell people your goals.

● Pace yourself—little and often is just as good as one strenuous session.

● Understand that exercise does not cure arthritis and episodes of pain are not necessarily related to exercising.

Neck exercises

Head turns, head rolls, and neck stretches (tilting your head from side to side) are simple exercises that you can do to improve the movement of your head on your shoulders. Before you start make sure you are standing—or sitting—straight and tall. Imagine that a string, connected to the top of your head, is holding you up and extending your neck. Keep your shoulders and upper limbs relaxed at all times. Breathe in through your nose and out through your mouth, slowly and gently.

HEAD TURNS

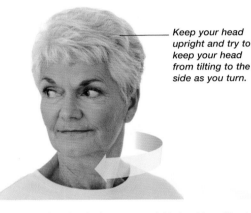

Keep your head upright and try to keep your head from tilting to the side as you turn.

Slowly turn your head to look over your right shoulder without tilting it to the side. Feel a gentle stretch and tightness in your neck. Breathe gently. Hold the position for 5 or 6 seconds.

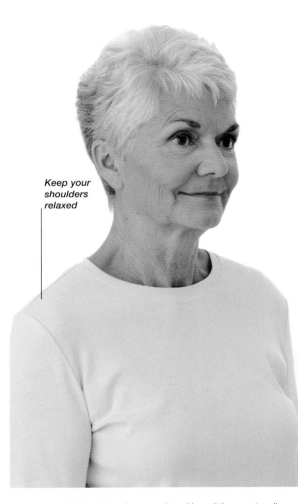

Keep your shoulders relaxed

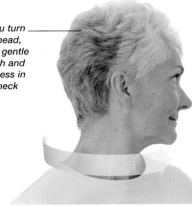

As you turn your head, feel a gentle stretch and tightness in your neck

You can do this head turning exercise either sitting or standing. If you are standing, make sure you are next to a wall or something to grab on to just in case you feel dizzy.

Now turn to look over your left shoulder, again without tilting your head to the side. Hold the position for 5 or 6 seconds. Repeat the full exercise sequence 5 or 6 times.

HEAD ROLLS

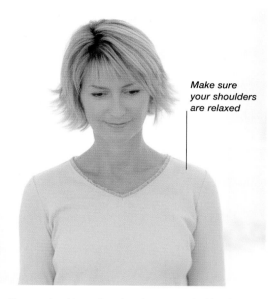

*Make sure
your shoulders
are relaxed*

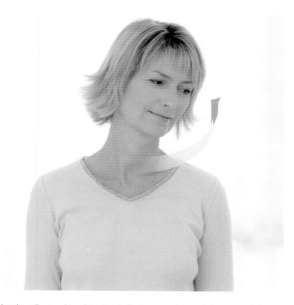

Start with your shoulders relaxed and your eyes looking forward. Slowly let your head fall to the front so that your chin drops down toward your chest and you are looking at the floor.

Slowly roll your head to the left. As you do so, bring your left ear as close to your left shoulder as you comfortably can, with your eyes looking in the direction your head is moving.

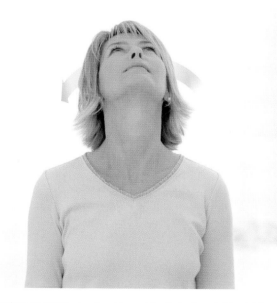

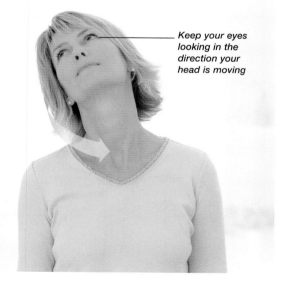

*Keep your eyes
looking in the
direction your
head is moving*

Continue to move your head in a wide circle, from left to right. When you reach midway, look upward toward the ceiling and feel a gentle stretch in the muscles in the front of your neck.

Come down with your right ear as close to your right shoulder as you comfortably can. Relax. Repeat 3 or 4 circles. Repeat the whole sequence, this time circling to the right.

Shoulder exercises

These three exercises are excellent for improving the range of movement in your shoulders. The windmill is particularly good for helping the ball-and-socket joint in your shoulders reach their fullest extent in any direction.

Each of the exercises will strengthen the shoulder joints and the muscles surrounding them, which will help you cope better with everyday tasks such as putting on your clothes, brushing your hair, driving, cleaning, and gardening.

WINDMILLS

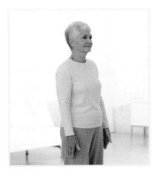

Stand relaxed with your arms by your sides. Slowly raise your arms up in front of you until you are reaching upward. Slowly lower them to the side and behind you. Relax. Repeat 5 or 6 circles.

Raise your arms up in front of you

Lower your arms to the side and behind you

Reverse the direction of the circle, going up behind and to the side, and lowering your arms in front of you.

SHOULDER ROTATION

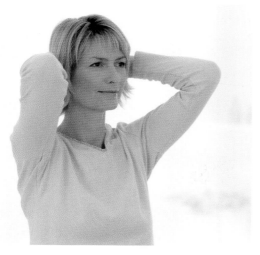 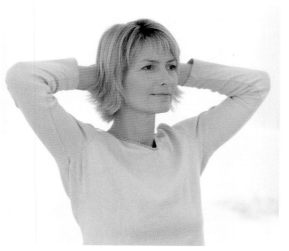

Clasp your hands behind your head, with your fingers interlocked. If you can't reach behind your head because it is uncomfortable, just place your hands as far back on the top of your head as you can. Gently push your elbows outward—but only within your comfort zone. Feel a gentle stretch under your arms beneath the shoulders. Hold this position for 5 seconds if you can. Exhale. Bring your forearms back close to your ears. Repeat the exercise 5 or 6 times.

"BACK DRY"

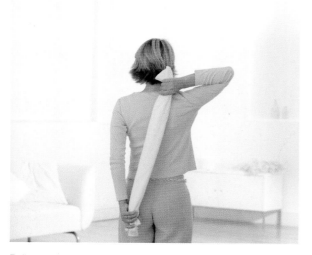 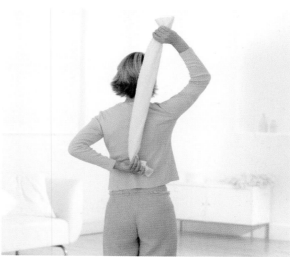

Roll up a small towel and grasp it as if you were drying your back—your right arm over the top of your right shoulder and your left arm in the small of your back. With your left hand gently pull the towel down, feeling a gentle pull in your right arm. Hold for 5 or 6 seconds. Now pull the towel up with your right hand and feel a gentle pull in your left arm. Hold for 5 or 6 seconds. Repeat the exercise 10 times. Then swap your hands—the left above your left shoulder and your right in the small of your back.

Back exercises

The sit-ups and easy push-ups are two of the many exercises that can help you with the flexibility of your lower back. If you have a pain in your lower back, consult your physician or physical therapist before trying these exercises.

Both exercises involve you lying down—if you use the floor, spread out a mat or towel to make it a little more comfortable. If you have difficulty bending down, take time to get into position and relax for a few minutes before starting.

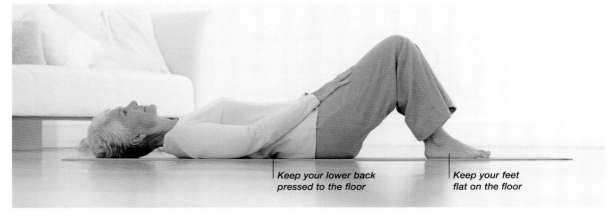

Keep your lower back pressed to the floor

Keep your feet flat on the floor

This exercise is designed to strengthen the muscles in your abdomen, which are important for the mobility of your back. Lie down on your back on the floor (or on a bed) with your knees bent and place your hands on your thighs. Relax your shoulders and let them sink toward the floor. Become conscious of your breathing as you inhale and exhale from your abdomen.

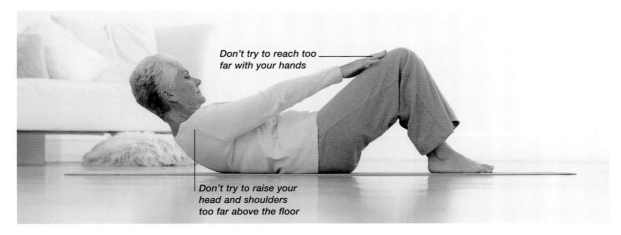

Don't try to reach too far with your hands

Don't try to raise your head and shoulders too far above the floor

Slowly run your hands up your thighs toward your knees, gently raising your head and shoulders off the floor. Don't reach too far. If you can, hold the position for 5 or 6 seconds, then exhale.

Relax as you roll down slowly. Rest for 5 or 6 seconds. Repeat the exercise 5 or 6 times. Over a few weeks increase the number of sit-ups and hold them for a little bit longer.

EASY PUSH-UPS

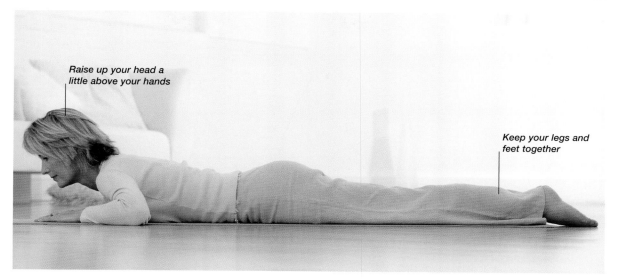

Raise up your head a little above your hands

Keep your legs and feet together

This exercise increases the mobility of the spine in your lower back and also the sacroiliac joints where the spine meets the pelvis. Lie face down on a mat or towel on the floor, with your elbows pointing out to the side and your hands placed flat on the floor under your shoulders. Relax your whole body and breathe gently. Raise your head.

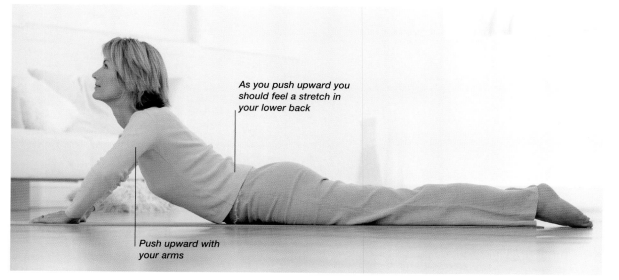

As you push upward you should feel a stretch in your lower back

Push upward with your arms

Inhale and hold in your breath as you push up with your arms and slowly straighten your elbows. Lift up your head and shoulders as high as you can within your comfort zone. Look up at the ceiling and, as you feel a stretch in region of your lower back, exhale. Feel your lower back sag slightly as you exhale. Hold this position for 5 or 6 seconds. Let your arms relax as they allow the trunk of your body to lower slowly to the floor. Repeat the exercise 5 or 6 times.

Leg and hip exercises

The following exercises will help people whether or not they have arthritis improve and maintain the mobility in their hips and knees. They help ease any stiffness and build up strength in the muscles surrounding the joints.

People with osteoarthritis of the knee or hip should obtain particular benefit from the step-ups and the sit-to-stand exercises. Make sure you always work within your comfort zone and avoid overstretching yourself.

STEP-UPS

Keep your head still and look ahead

Hold on to give yourself support

Raise your left leg and step up

Step up and down with your right foot

Place your left foot on a low, stable step (e.g. the bottom stair or pile of 3 telephone directories). Hold on to the banisters, wall, or chair for support. Keeping your left foot on the step, step up and down with your right foot for a minute. Repeat 5 or 6 times,

resting for short time between each. Put your right foot on the step and repeat the exercise. As you gradually increase the number of step-ups, raise the height of the step (making sure you are stable and safe) to a maximum of about 18in (45cm).

GENTLE SQUATS

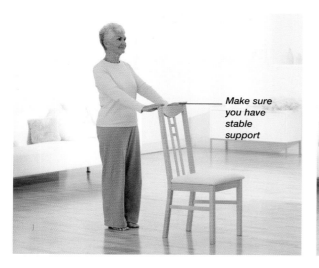

Make sure you have stable support

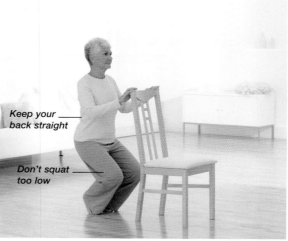

Keep your back straight

Don't squat too low

Stand upright with your feet flat on the floor and look straight ahead. Gently steady yourself by resting your hands on a stable object (such as the back of a chair) positioned in front of you. Keeping your back straight, slowly bend your knees into a gentle squat and then straighten your knees until you are standing again. Repeat 10 times. As you improve, squat down a little further, but not beyond 90 degrees and never squat fully because it puts great strain on your knees.

HIP ROTATIONS

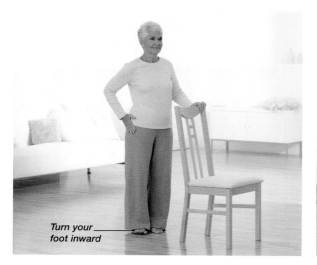

Turn your foot inward

Turn your foot outward

Stand upright with one hand resting on a stable object, such as the back of a chair. Place your right hand on the front of your right hip and hitch up the hip so that your right foot is an inch or two off the ground. Turn your foot inward to the left as far as it will go (feel your hip turning inward under your hand). Hold the position for 5 or 6 seconds. Turn your foot outward to the right (again feeling your hip turn) and hold for 5 or 6 seconds. Repeat the sequence 10 times. Then repeat with the left foot 10 times.

LEG STRENGTHENING

Tie an elastic inner tube of a
bicycle tire or a commercially
available resistive exercise
band (e.g. Thera-Band™)
to an immovable object, such
as the leg of a chair or bed.
Loop it around your right foot.

*Sit upright
with your
back straight
and your
head still*

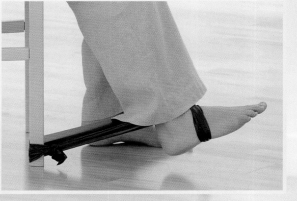

Sit upright on the chair and slowly
straighten your knee as far as you can,
stretching the band. Hold the position for
5 seconds. The tension in the band will
pull your leg back to the starting position.
It is important that you control this return
and make sure it is slow. Repeat for
1–2 minutes. Repeat using your left foot.

As you improve, perform the exercise
for longer, hold your leg straight for
longer, and/or increase the resistance
by making the loop smaller or using
a stiffer resistive band.

*Tie the elastic band to
a chair leg and loop it
around your foot*

SIT-TO-STANDS

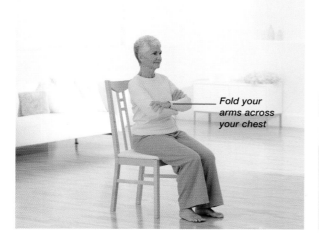

Fold your arms across your chest

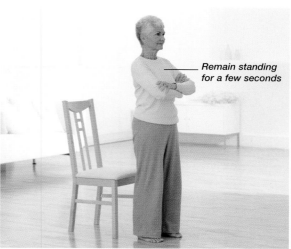

Remain standing for a few seconds

Sit upright on a chair, looking straight ahead, your feet flat on the ground, and your arms folded across your chest. Stand up slowly without using your arms and remain in the standing position for a few seconds. Sit down slowly. Continue to do these sit-to-stands for about a minute. Over a period of a few weeks, try to increase the number of sit-to-stands you do—or start from a lower chair or the next-to-bottom stair. Never strain yourself and always make sure you are in control.

KNEE FLEXIONS

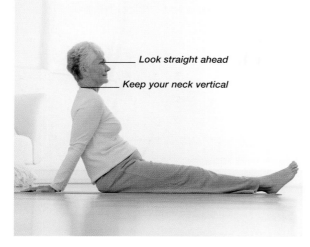

Look straight ahead

Keep your neck vertical

You should feel a comfortable stretch in your leg

Hold position for 5–6 seconds

Sit on the floor, couch, or bed with your legs together and stretched out in front of you. Place your hands on the floor behind you so that they take the weight of your upper body. Keep your neck vertical and look straight ahead.

Slowly move your right knee toward you until it is bent and you can feel a comfortable stretch. Hold this position for 5 or 6 seconds before straightening your leg again. Rest for 3 seconds. Repeat the sequence 10 times. Repeat using your left leg.

TRUNK ROTATIONS

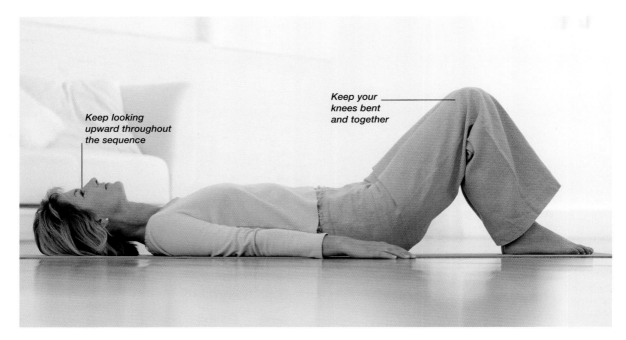

Keep looking upward throughout the sequence

Keep your knees bent and together

Lie on the floor or a bed with knees bent, shoulders relaxed, arms beside you, and look upward. Slowly let your knees fall to the right, keeping them together as you do so and still looking up (below). Stop when you feel a gentle stretch in your lower back and left thigh, and hold the position for 5 or 6 seconds.

Return to the starting position. Now repeat the exercise, this time letting your knees fall gently to the left (below) and holding for 5 or 6 seconds. Repeat the whole sequence 10 times. Rest for 30 seconds. Repeat 5 times. Over a few weeks as your trunk loosens up, let your knees to fall slightly further to the sides.

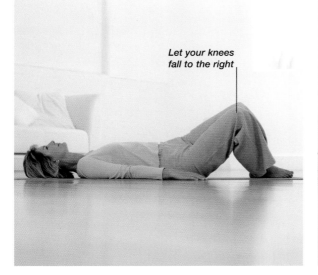

Let your knees fall to the right

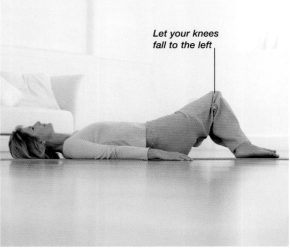

Let your knees fall to the left

HIP EXTENSIONS

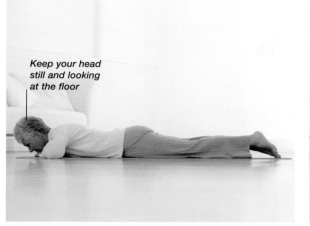

Keep your head still and looking at the floor

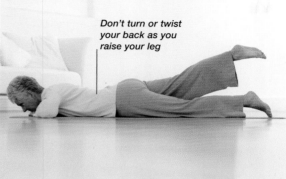

Don't turn or twist your back as you raise your leg

Lie comfortably on your front on a mat on the floor (or on a bed) so that you are resting your chin on your hands. Without turning or twisting your back, slowly raise your right leg up behind you about 3–4in (7.5–10cm). Hold this position for 4 to 5 seconds if you can before slowly lowering your leg to the floor. Relax your body and exhale. Repeat 5 times. Repeat with left leg. As you improve, try to raise each leg a little higher, hold it up a little longer, and/or increase the number of leg raises.

HIP ABDUCTIONS

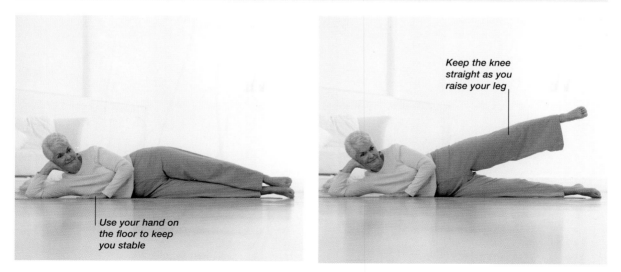

Use your hand on the floor to keep you stable

Keep the knee straight as you raise your leg

Lie comfortably on your right side on a mat on the floor (or on a bed) and prop up your head with your right hand. Keeping your left knee straight, slowly raise your left leg into the air—about 2ft (60cm) if you can. Hold the position for 5 or 6 seconds, then slowly lower the leg, and relax. Repeat 10 times. Turn over and repeat the exercise with your right leg. As you improve, increase the number of lifts, raise each leg a little higher, and hold it for a little longer. Make sure the movements are slow and controlled.

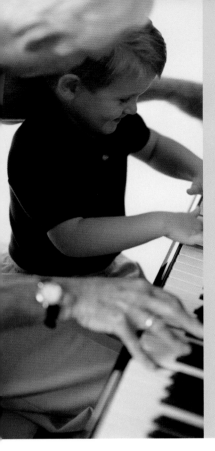

Protecting your joints

Joints and muscles have to last a lifetime, so taking care of them makes sense. Some of the ways of protecting your joints were developed in the workplace to reduce the strain on workers. You may already be doing some of them, while others can be hard to accept at first. Once you use the methods often enough in your daily life, you will reap the benefits. You will have less pain and fatigue, and will find doing jobs easier and less frustrating—and you'll have energy left over so you can enjoy life more.

Protecting your joints is not about giving up activities —just finding easier ways of doing them.

Why protect your joints?

How you stand and move your body affects the stress and strain you place upon your joints. For example, a slouched posture increases the stress on your back and neck. You will put strain on your muscles and joints if you repeat the same movement over and over, or if you hold a joint in the same restricted position for too long. Even using too much effort to do a job can be stressful.

We all develop movement habits that may not be the most efficient. But when you have arthritis this inefficiency increases your fatigue and adds to your pain.

Straining swollen and painful joints can further weaken their support structures (ligaments, tendons, and joint capsules). In time, deformities may develop. Straining muscles increases fatigue.

If it hurts, change it
Protecting your joints does not require that you give up activities —just finding easier ways of doing them. Most people develop their own ways to reduce pain and fatigue over the years. But it takes time to work out solutions for yourself. People with arthritis

often get used to pain, and medication can mask it, so you may not notice that an activity causes strain, pain, or fatigue until afterward. Then you regret overdoing it the next day. So the rule is: if it hurts, change it.

Shortcuts to making changes

The ideas in this chapter will help you take shortcuts to making the kind of changes that will keep your muscles and joints as healthy as possible. The sooner you make the changes, the better for your joints in the long run. Making activities easier will not weaken your muscles—they will reduce your fatigue and pain, leaving you more energy to exercise. The chapters on physical activity and mobility (see pp.64–73 and pp.158–171) show you how to move your joints fully and strengthen your muscles.

Changing your habits

Arthritis can cause some joints to deform over time. For example, if you have rheumatoid arthritis your wrists can start to move downward and your fingers point away from the thumb. In thumb osteoarthritis, a zigzag shape can develop.

Many activities, such as lifting, can put a downward pressure or pull on the wrist. Others, such as opening a jar or turning faucets,

require twisting movements at the knuckles. Over time, this weakens ligaments and joints start to move in the direction of the pressure.

Look at how you move your joints and muscles and see if you can find a way of doing it differently, applying the seven principles on p.174. Changing habits may be challenging at first since the old ones are ingrained. Once you get used to analyzing what you are doing, the ideas will start to snowball.

A step-by-step technique

Start changing your habits in a step-by-step way. Pick a common daily activity, such as making a cup of tea. Watch how you use your hands and the joints and muscles that cause you pain.

Check to see how you hold your joints while moving and working. For example, are your wrists bent

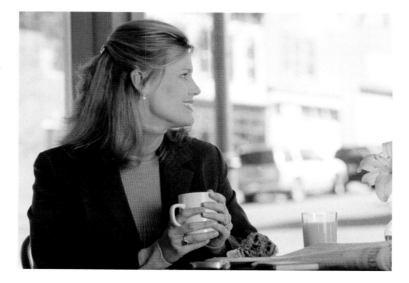

HOLDING A CUP
When you drink a cup of tea or coffee, try holding the cup with both hands rather than putting strain on the fingers of one hand.

sideways or downward rather than in a straight line or upright? Is there hard pressure on the ends of your fingers and thumbs? Are you gripping too tightly?

If you answer yes to these questions, how can you change the movement or activity to make it easier? Think about the seven principles below and write down your solutions in a diary. Practice this technique as often as you can over the next week or two.

Key principles to protect your joints

The following seven key principles use biomechanics and ergonomics to help you protect your joints and manage your fatigue:

● Use your larger, stronger muscles and joints.

● Spread the load over several of your joints.
● Avoid twisting actions.
● Use the least effort.
● Avoid staying in the same position for too long.
● Plan your activities more efficiently.
● Pace your activities.

Biomechanics involves the use of efficient physical techniques for standing, sitting, walking, and bending, as well as for lifting and handling objects. Ergonomics involves the design of tasks and equipment that fit a person's abilities to their activities and to their environment in the most effective way possible.

Use your larger, stronger muscles and joints

Don't put pressure on your small joints and muscles when your larger, stronger ones can do a job more effectively. For example, if you have hand problems you can carry bags over your forearm or shoulder (or use a backpack if you can). Another example is to use your thigh muscles and elbows to push up out of a chair rather than pushing down with your knuckles.

Avoid twisting actions

Twisting actions that use force can cause pain and discomfort. For example, rather than using your fingers to twist a tight lid off a jar, press down on it with the palm of the hand or hold the lid of the jar

OPENING A JAR
The best way to unscrew the lid of a jar is to press down with your palm or hold the side of the jar lid between the curve of your thumb and fingers. Then unscrew the lid with your arm.

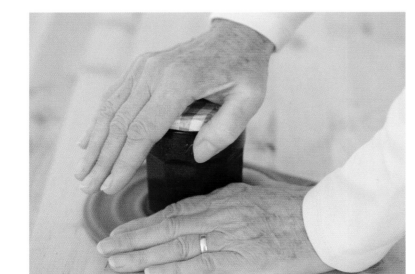

lid between the curve of your thumb and fingers. A small non-slip mat or a jar opener (available in kitchen stores) can also help.

If you have hip, knee, or foot problems, get up from a chair with your weight spread over both legs, rather than leaning to one side.

Spread the load over several of your joints

Don't rely on one joint to do a job when several joints can share the load. For example, use the palms of both hands to lift things. Hold pots in both palms, rather than with fingers and thumbs—it also reduces the risk of dropping things.

When pouring water from a hot tea kettle, grip the handle with one hand while the palm of the other supports the side of the kettle with a potholder. Using two hands in this way cuts the strain on each wrist and hand by 50 percent.

Use the least effort

There are several ways to minimize the effort you use to accomplish various tasks:

■ **DON'T GRIP OBJECTS TOO TIGHTLY** If you have hand problems, use kitchen gadgets and household and home repair tools with nonslip handles so that you don't have to grip as hard. You can also pad out normal handles slightly— for example, with foam tubing from a home maintenance store. To help you write, use a thicker pen or a pen grip (see p.139).

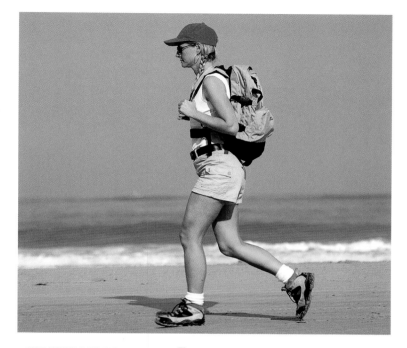

SPREAD THE LOAD
Using a backpack is a good example of spreading the load and letting the larger, stronger muscles take the strain.

■ **USE WHEELS TO MOVE OBJECTS** For example, use a shopping cart to move laundry around your house or to the laundromat, or to move the shopping from the car to the house. Use a briefcase or backpack with wheels and an extendable handle to carry your laptop and office papers.

■ **USE ASSISTIVE DEVICES** See p.140 for some of the many readily available assistive devices.

■ **USE LABOR-SAVING EQUIPMENT** Consider buying labor-saving household equipment, such as a clothes drier and a dishwasher. The money is well spent if the equipment reduces your fatigue and pain, and gives you more energy and time to spend with your family and friends, and on activities you enjoy.

TASK ANALYSIS: IRONING

Task analysis is a technique used in industry and management that can also help you with domestic jobs. It enables you to focus on ways of protecting your joints so that you do the job with less stress and a minimum of effort. Ironing is an example of how you could use task analysis for a common household job.

PROBLEM	POSSIBLE SOLUTION
Amount of ironing	• Keep the amount of ironing to a minimum. Buy easy-care or permanent-press items. Hang up clothes straight after drying to avoid wrinkles. • Ask yourself if you really need to iron the item.
Ironing board	• Leave the ironing board up, attach a drop-down board to a wall, or buy a lightweight board. • Use a board with a metal stand to lay the iron flat. Up-ending the iron strains your wrist. • Use a reflective board cover so you don't have to iron both sides of an item.
Iron	• Attach a pull to the plug to make plugging and unplugging easy. • Use a lightweight iron with a long cord, a good grip surface to the handle, and a toggle switch to turn the steam function on and off.
Doing the ironing	• "Little and often" are the key watch words. • Use an ironing stool to take the weight off your legs. Move around regularly. Take microbreaks. • Wear a wrist splint. • Keep the weight of the iron to a minimum—do the items that need steaming last so that you just put water in when you need it.

Avoid staying in the same position for too long

Whenever you feel as though you're sitting or standing in the same position for a long time, change it. If you're in a sitting position, get up and move around for a minute or two every half-hour. Alternatively, stretch your legs out and move your ankles every few minutes.

Take regular microbreaks too (see right). This is particularly important if you work at a computer or in a job where you sit or stand in a similar position for long periods.

Balance your heavier and lighter activities. For example, swap vacuuming with dusting, or lawn mowing with light weeding every 15 minutes or so. If you have hand problems, swap repetitive tasks—for example, chopping, cutting, or stirring when cooking, or weeding, pruning, and digging when gardening.

This swapping around of tasks will help you avoid using the same muscle groups in the same repetitive patterns, or continually overworking them for too long. Your joints also get a regular change of position.

Plan your activities more efficiently

Most people have a habitual way of carrying out their regular daily activities. They rarely ask if they can be done more efficiently. If you are in a hurry, you often make more mistakes and waste time—as well as creating more muscle tension and fatigue.

Take the time to plan ahead. For each of the domestic activities you need to do, try out the following task analysis approach (see left, for the example of ironing):

Q&A

"Will planning and pacing my activities mean that I'm giving in and make me weaker?"

No. Research shows that those who do best in the long term are those who believe they can manage their condition effectively. Look for solutions that help you cope positively and try to avoid getting frustrated. You can save energy by planning and pacing yourself—then you will have more energy for doing the things you enjoy.

• What steps and different tasks are involved in doing the activity?
• In what order can these steps or tasks be done most efficiently?
• Could you make the activity simpler? Or cut down on the amount that needs to be done?
• Could you do the activity by moving differently or by using differently designed pieces of equipment—for example, one with wheels?
• Would wearing a splint, such as a wrist splint or knee brace, help reduce the effort required?
• What is the best body position to use when doing the activity?
• Is everything you need right by you? If the answer is yes, you will reduce the number of trips around the house or office (or across a room) to collect what you need to do the job.
• Are the items you need stored efficiently? Items regularly used for the same tasks should be stored

near one another. Keep items near the place where they are most frequently used. Arrange your organizers such as drawer dividers, cabinet shelves, both fixed and adjustable, so that you can easily reach and pick up items.

Pace your activities

Think of yourself as a battery with a fixed amount of energy for the day. Spend it wisely on what you both need and want to do. Life is about enjoying yourself so it is important for your health to give yourself time for leisure and social activities. Regular rests and breaks act as battery rechargers and regular changes of activity will ease muscle tension.

Balance periods of rest and activity. Take a regular break for a few minutes every 30–45 minutes. If you cannot do this, at least take a break for 15 minutes every 2 hours. Sit and let your neck and shoulder muscles relax and let the tension ease away.

Perhaps you think you don't have time to take a rest, or that having a rest means that you are giving in to your arthritis. However, your body will need a longer recovery time if you work for long periods without a break. Research shows that people who take regular short breaks and microbreaks are active for longer, more productive, and less tired by the end of the day. Allow yourself to take a break. It's healthier.

Regular rests and breaks act as battery rechargers and regular changes of activity will ease muscle tension.

PRACTICAL TIPS

TAKING MICROBREAKS

Train yourself to take small, regular breaks from whatever you are doing.

• Every 5–10 minutes stretch the joints and muscles you are using for 30–60 seconds.

• Try to move around every 15–30 minutes or so.

• Set up an alarm on your computer, kitchen timer, or cell phone (or set this to vibrate if you don't want to annoy others) to remind yourself to take microbreaks. After a few days you will find that the habit of taking breaks starts to form.

WORKING AT A COMPUTER

When you work at a computer, the following advice will help you adopt the best posture so that your joints and muscles do not experience too much stress and strain.

● Buy an ergonomic chair so you can adjust its height. Your knees and the chair must go under the desk to help you sit with your hips at right angles and your back supported.

● Raise the seat or lower the keyboard so you can sit with your shoulders relaxed, elbows comfortably bent, and wrists straight on the keyboard.

● Place the screen at eye level to avoid bending your neck. Voice activation software may help.

● Use an ergonomic keyboard and mouse. If you need to write, clear the desk space rather than leaning awkwardly to one side.

● Don't rest your wrists on the desk edge—use a wrist rest.

● Take microbreaks every 5–10 minutes. Stretch muscles and relax your shoulders and neck.

● Don't clutter your desk area.

● Regular phone users could buy a hands-free phone or headset to avoid leaning to one side.

REDUCE THE STRAIN
Setting up your computer, desk, and chair so that your body is comfortable and not awkward reduces the strain on your joints.

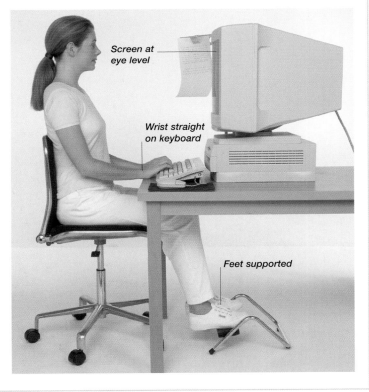

Screen at eye level

Wrist straight on keyboard

Feet supported

Posture

Proper body alignment uses less energy because your weight is balanced centrally. The three curves to the spine—a slight forward curve at the neck, a backward curve at the mid-back, and a forward curve in the lumbar region—help absorb shocks when you move.

Poor posture increases muscle tension and pain in your neck, shoulder, and lower back. There are two common problems: sitting or standing with your head poked forward, shoulders hunched, and the lower back slumped; and standing with your knees locked, which arches the lower back and pushes the head forward.

Standing posture

When you stand, keep your ears in line with your shoulders, which should be relaxed and in line with your hips. Keep your hips in line with your knees and ankles, with your knees very slightly relaxed (not locked rigid) and your weight evenly distributed over your feet.

Sitting posture

When you sit, keep your head upright with your ears over your relaxed shoulders. Relax your upper back and keep it over your hips. Make sure your hips and knees are at right angles (check that your seat is not too low). Evenly distribute your weight

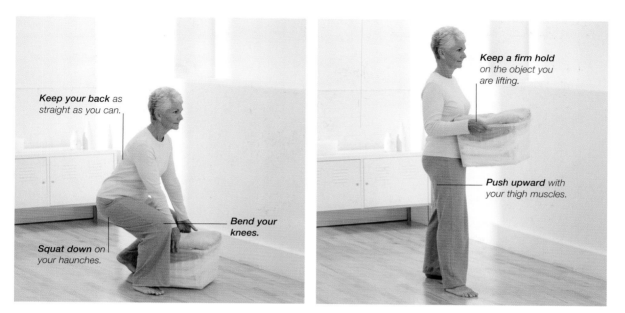

GETTING INTO POSITION
If you have to lift a moderately heavy object, first make sure that you get close to it—then squat down on your haunches and bend your knees rather than your back.

LIFTING THE OBJECT
Make sure you have a firm hold on the object. Tighten your stomach muscles. Keep the weight close to your body and push upward using your thigh muscles rather than your back muscles.

Keep your back as straight as you can.

Squat down on your haunches.

Bend your knees.

Keep a firm hold on the object you are lifting.

Push upward with your thigh muscles.

across your bottom (not leaning to one side), and make sure your bottom is to the back of chair seat so your back is supported. Finally, put your feet flat on the floor.

You spend considerable part of the day sitting down, so you should make sure that your chairs and sofa are good quality. Poor-quality furniture and a slumped posture put extra strain on your joints and back (see right).

Moving and lifting
Avoid moving and lifting heavy objects. There are safe ways to lift moderately heavy items (see above). If you have to lift objects as part of your job, your employer

is required by law to provide you with training and equipment to make this easier.

Walking
Invest in a pair of good shoes for walking (see p.70). These should have shock-absorbing soles or insoles, a continuous sole with a slightly beveled heel, and firm support over the top of the foot (either laces or straps).

Many people with foot and leg problems habitually look down at the ground in front of their feet when walking because they are worried about tripping. Train yourself to look ahead a few yards to help with your posture.

PRACTICAL TIPS

SEATING CHECKPOINTS
● Your chair or sofa should have a firm seat. Put a board under a saggy sofa seat and change the seat cushion for firmer foam.

● The height of your seat should allow you to sit so that your hips and knees are at right angles.

● Make sure you have a supportive back rest— preferably up to shoulder and head height so that you can relax your head and neck. Check that you have good back support—use a small cushion if it helps.

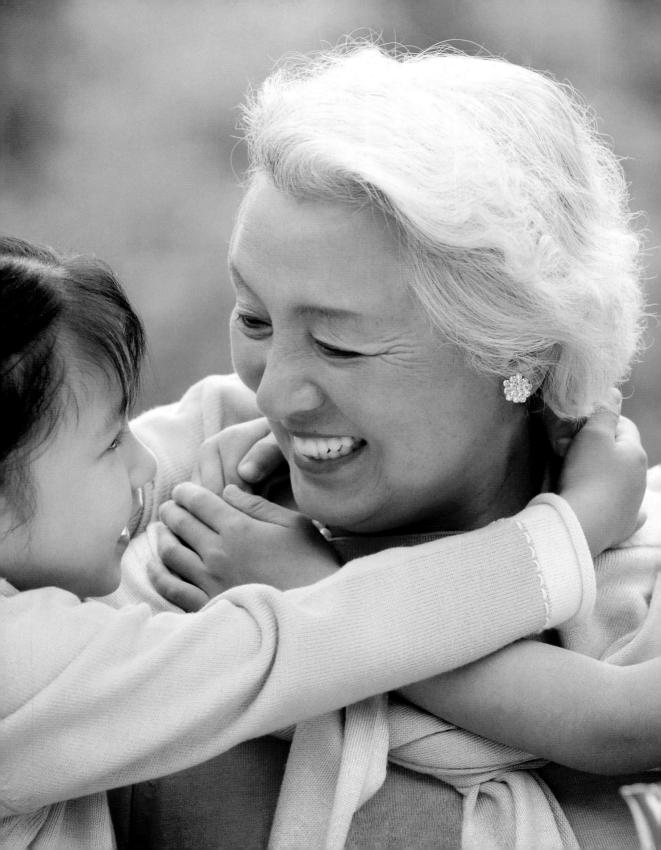

Children and special risk groups

For a long time, people thought arthritis was a condition that primarily affected elderly people. This perception is gradually changing as it becomes clear that arthritis affects other parts of the population in significant numbers.

Arthritis in children can be hard to detect but often develops in a similar way to arthritis in adults. What is different is that children have special needs that must be addressed for them to grow up as normally as possible.

Foremost among the groups at special risk are postmenopausal women, who are prone to arthritis and osteoporosis. Managing menopause with hormone replacements can help but brings risks of its own.

Obesity and excessive physical activity that puts joints under repeated strain increases the risk of osteoarthritis—a risk that is reduced by losing weight and ceasing the repeated activity. People who inherit a predisposition to arthritis can expect to benefit from improved medication and advances in surgical treatments.

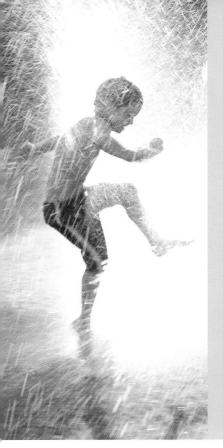

Arthritis in children

Few people realize that arthritis affects children as well as adults. In fact, juvenile arthritis seems to catch everyone by surprise, probably because it is easy to overlook and difficult to diagnose. It may take months or years to confirm a diagnosis of arthritis in a child, let alone start effective treatment. However, children with arthritis can benefit from all kinds of therapeutic care and support, while at the same time receiving help for their special needs—at school, home, and at play.

If your child experiences pain in one or more joints he or she may not necessarily have arthritis.

Types of childhood arthritis

Each year, arthritis will affect approximately one child in every thousand. Most of these cases are generally mild and self-limiting (that is, they do not get worse over time). More severe types of arthritis affect approximately one child in every 10,000.

Juvenile arthritis is the classic example of inflammatory arthritis occurring in children. However, reactive arthritis, septic arthritis, and some other forms of adult arthritis (see pp.14–22) can also affect children.

Juvenile arthritis

Between 30,000 and 50,000 children in the US are affected by juvenile arthritis. Also known as juvenile idiopathic or juvenile rheumatoid arthritis, it involves pain, inflammation, and swelling in at least one joint. It may run in families and seems to result from an abnormal immune response.

Depending on the joints involved in the early months of disease and the involvement of other organs, juvenile arthritis is divided into five main types:

■ **OLIGOARTICULAR JUVENILE ARTHRITIS** At the start less than four joints are involved. This type accounts for about half of the cases of juvenile arthritis. A young child (perhaps as young as 2 or 3 years of age) may have a swollen knee or ankle, which appears without injury or explanation.

Often, the arthritis is mild but may be associated with uveitis. This condition, in which the eyes become inflamed, is not necessarily painful but it may result in scarring and permanent damage to the child's eyesight if left untreated.

■ **POLYARTHRITIS** At least 5 joints are involved from the start in this type, which accounts for 40 percent of the cases of juvenile arthritis. It can begin in children of any age, even just a few months.It is similar to adult rheumatoid arthritis. Some children with polyarthritis test positive for rheumatoid factor (see p.184). Polyarthritis, especially with a positive rheumatoid factor, causes more joint damage than oligoarthritis.

Q&A

"Can children with juvenile arthritis develop osteoporosis?"

Yes. Children who have been badly affected by juvenile arthritis can later develop osteoporosis (see p.35). DXA (dual energy X-ray absorptiometry) scans may be used to identify it early if physicians are concerned. Calcium and vitamin D supplements are prescribed, and bisphosphonates considered if the child is on corticosteroids such as prednisone.

■ **SYSTEMIC ARTHRITIS** This type accounts for 10 percent of cases. It often starts with a rash and high fever, which varies throughout the day and is often absent for many hours. The disease may vanish without returning, or the fever and rash clears up, but the arthritis progresses and can become severe. It may involve the internal organs and, rarely, can be life threatening.

■ **ENTHESITIS-RELATED ARTHRITIS** This type involves the spine, hips, and the entheses (the points where tendons attach to bones). It mainly affects boys over 8 years of age.

■ **PSORIATRIC ARTHRITIS** In this type children have both arthritis and psoriasis. It is similar to psoriatric arthritis in adults (see p.22).

Other causes of joint pain

If your child experiences pain in one or more joints he or she may not necessarily have arthritis. The pain might be due to a condition that affects the mechanical way the joint works or to a chronic pain syndrome of unknown cause, such as fibromyalgia (see p.27).

Several different diseases can cause mechanical problems. Some are rare inherited disorders that involve the protein collagen or another part of the connective tissue. Others are blood problems, such as sickle-cell disease, or musculoskeletal problems, such as Osgood Schlatter's disease, which causes inflammation and pain in front of the shinbone (tibia).

Juvenile arthritis sometimes runs in families and seems to result from an abnormal immune response.

Occasionally, children with leukemia develop symptoms that are very similar to the onset of childhood arthritis. An arthritic kind of joint pain may be a feature of inflammatory bowel disease, such as Crohn's disease.

Rheumatic fever may cause a type of arthritis involving several, or even many, joints. However, this is rare and occurs in less than 1 in 100,000 children in industrialized countries.

Signs to look out for

Arthritis may be hard to diagnose in a child and the first features can be very nonspecific. For example, the child may be generally unwell or complain of pain.

Arthritis changes the way a child walks or uses his or her arms, legs, hands, and feet. Pain often limits the movement of an affected joint, although younger children may not complain of pain. If joints in the legs are involved the child may start to limp or walk with difficulty.

Another sign is swelling in a child's joint, particularly when accompanied by pain and stiffness. Stiffness is especially worrisome when it persists, or is worse in the morning or after a nap.

BLOOD TESTS

In general, blood tests for children who may or may not have arthritis are the same tests as those for an adult. They analyze the cell content of the blood—red blood cells, white blood cells, and platelets—and measure the erythrocyte sedimentation rate (ESR) and the levels of auto-antibodies, such as rheumatoid factor, and antinuclear antibodies (see p.41).

BLOOD TEST	REASON FOR TEST
Blood count	To measure the level of hemoglobin—low levels may indicate anemia, a blood disorder that might have a link to arthritis. High levels of white blood cells and blood platelets may indicate infection or inflammation.
Liver function	To measure the level of some enzymes to check the liver is working properly and to see if it can deal with drugs such as methotrexate.
Kidney function	To measure the level of waste products and salts to check that the kidneys are working properly.
Erythrocyte sedimentation rate test (see p.41)	To assess the body's response to a damaging situation, such as inflammation or infection.
Auto-antibodies	To look for auto-antibodies, such as rheumatoid factor and antinuclear antibodies. These may be able to help diagnose the different types of juvenile idiopathic arthritis.
C-reactive protein test (CRP)	To measure the level of C-reactive protein, which is a protein produced by the liver when there is acute inflammation.

Diagnosis

If your doctor suspects that your child has arthritis, he or she will arrange for some blood tests (see left) and some imaging studies to help confirm a diagnosis.

Blood tests

Just as with adults, a positive result for any blood test does not necessarily confirm a diagnosis of arthritis. Many children with juvenile arthritis have neither rheumatoid factor nor antinuclear

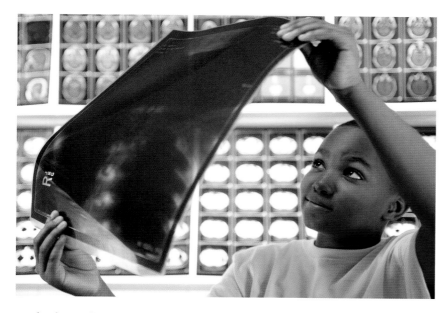

IMAGES OF JOINTS
X-rays and MRI scans can help doctors to look closely at joints to see if they are damaged or swollen.

antibodies. Also, many children with conditions other than arthritis can have either rheumatoid factor or antinuclear antibodies.

Nevertheless, the presence of either antinuclear antibodies or rheumatoid factor is highly suggestive of juvenile arthritis. A quarter of children with arthritis, especially oligoarthritis, test positive for antinuclear antibodies. Rheumatoid factor usually indicates polyarthritis that will continue into adult life.

Systemic arthritis is accompanied by a high ESR reading (see p.41). It is usually high in polyarthritis, too, but often normal in oligoarthritis.

Taking images

To help confirm a diagnosis or assess the severity of arthritis, your child may need X-rays or, rarely, a magnetic resonance imaging (MRI) scan, to show the extent of joint damage. They can identify the presence of bone erosions in one or more joints or show the presence of excessive fluid within a joint.

Managing a child's arthritis

In some areas a dedicated pediatric rheumatologist (a pediatrician specially trained in managing arthritis) will look after a child with arthritis.

In other areas, this role may be shared by a dedicated adult rheumatologist with a special interest in children and a general pediatrician. These highly qualified specialists are supported by physical therapists (see p.46) and occupational therapists (see p.144).

Arthritis may be hard to diagnose in a child because they frequently fight common illnesses and often lab tests are not diagnostic.

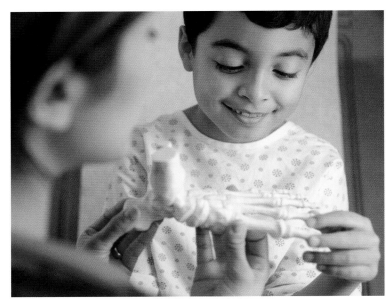

TALKING ABOUT JOINTS
Children with arthritis can enjoy finding out how their joints work.

The main goals of this care team are to manage your child's arthritis while simultaneously keeping the child in good physical condition and an active part of your family and community. To help the team achieve these goals, your child is treated to reduce swelling and pain, maintain the movement in affected joints, and prevent complications before they arise or resolve them when they do.

Nonsteroidal anti-inflammatory drugs

A few nonsteroidal anti-inflammatory drugs (NSAIDs), such as ibuprofen and naproxen, can be prescribed by your child's pediatrician. Childen are not usually treated with aspirin because it may cause bleeding problems, stomach upset, liver problems, or Reyes syndrome.

NSAIDs are effective in reducing pain and stiffness, but do not have any long-term impact on the disease. They may also cause multiple side-effects, particularly stomach problems and ulcers.

Disease-modifying anti-rheumatic drugs

When NSAIDs no longer relieve symptoms, or X-rays show bone damage, disease-modifying antirheumatic drugs (DMARDs) may be prescribed. These can relieve symptoms and slow the progress of juvenile idiopathic arthritis when it becomes a long-term illness. However, DMARDS take weeks or months to have an effect, so they are usually given with an NSAID.

The same DMARDs are used in children as in adults (see pp.83). Methotrexate is preferred, since the small doses needed to treat the disease do not usually cause potentially dangerous side effects. The most serious one is liver damage, which can be avoided by regular blood screening tests and careful follow-up. If a child develops a chest problem, such as a persistent dry cough, the methotrexate is discontinued due to the possibility of methotrexate lung disease.

Steroids

When a child's arthritis is severe and uncontrolled, or when the inflammation affects internal

Q&A

"Do children who are treated with steroids grow up to be shorter than normal adults?"

This is usually true. In one study, nearly half of adults with previous systemic juvenile idiopathic arthritis who were treated with steroids for at least 2 years during childhood had a final height that was substantially below their projected target height. More than 80 percent of the adults were shorter than anticipated.

organs, rheumatologists may add steroids such as prednisone to existing treatments. Steroids can be given by mouth or by injections into a vein (intravenously) or into the muscles (intramuscularly).

Steroids are very effective in the short term, but their effectiveness decreases over time. They have many potential side effects: they can interfere with normal growth; produce a red, round face; cause osteoporosis and diabetes; and increase susceptibility to infections.

Once steroids have started to control severe arthritis symptoms, the dose is gradually reduced and then stopped. Stopping steroids suddenly can be dangerous, so it is important to follow the dosing instructions very carefully.

Biologic agents

Children with severe polyarticular arthritis who have gained little relief from other drugs may be prescribed a biologic agent, such as etanercept (see p.85). Biologic agents are usually prescribed with DMARDs such as methotrexate, which rapidly improve symptoms and reduce inflammation.

DMARDs and biologic agents lower the immune response, increasing the risk of infections such as tuberculosis. As a result of the risks and high cost, biologic agents are prescribed with caution, usually after DMARDS have not been effective for at least 3 months.

Physical therapy

A key component of treatment is physical exercise supervised by a physical therapist, to help maintain muscle tone and preserve and recover joint movement. When the arthritis is severe, an occupational therapist may recommend splints (see p.138) to help maintain growth and reduce pain.

Steroids are very effective in the short term, but their effectiveness decreases over time.

SEEING A PHYSICAL THERAPIST
The expertise of a physical therapist can help children with arthritis improve muscle tone and maintain mobility in their joints.

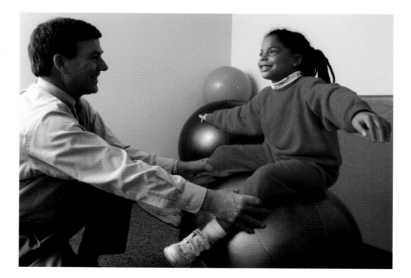

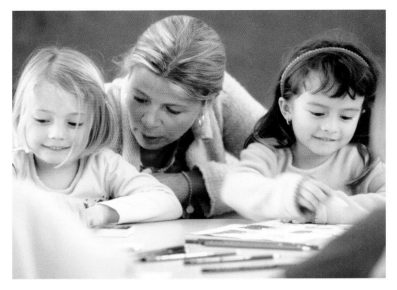

AT SCHOOL
Schoolteachers can help children with arthritis conserve energy so that they can concentrate their attention on their education.

Food and diet

Children with arthritis benefit from a healthy diet (see p.50) that includes protein, fruits, vegetables, calcium, and omega-3 fatty acids. They do not need a special diet or any extra vitamins or supplements, although, if taken in moderation, these will do no harm.

Complementary therapies

Children with arthritis should always be treated with conventional medicine. Some complementary approaches to health (see pp.108–125) may help a child cope with the stress of living with a chronic illness. However, they are not strongly supported by research evidence. Always ask your doctor for reassurance. If he or she considers a particular approach has value and will not cause harm, you can incorporate it into your child's treatment plan.

Special needs at school

Going to school is an essential part of every child's life and children with arthritis are no exception. It is important, therefore, that their parents, the clinicians involved in their care, and the teachers who educate them work closely together to make sure they receive the best possible education.

It is generally accepted that children with arthritis should remain within the normal school system. However, if your child's arthritis is severe and leads to hospitalization for any length of time, provisions should be made so his or her education can continue during that time.

Moving around

At school, your child may need special consideration because of difficulty writing (see opposite) or moving around as quickly as other children. Your child may need help to conserve as much energy as possible for schoolwork. Transportation to and from school is important, too, all the more so in the morning when joint stiffness can be acute. Going to school often means carrying around heavy bags, so ask for an extra locker or if your child can keep textbooks at home.

When your child is at school, moving quickly between classes can be difficult. Ask the teachers if they will let your child leave lessons a few minutes before other pupils. It may be impossible for schools to organize, but the ideal situation would be for children with arthritis to attend lessons on the ground floor in a reasonably small area that keeps walking distances short and avoids stairs.

Gaining confidence

Break times and PE lessons can be a challenge. Some active playtime and indoor activities with friends is essential to avoid feelings of isolation and to reduce stiffness.

However, children with active arthritis may be unable to exercise much and they often feel uncertain or embarrassed about their illness. Encourage your child to talk about his or her worries with a friend or a sympathetic teacher and so gain more confidence about joining in.

Special needs at play

Arthritis does not have to prevent a child from participating in active play, which is an essential part of growing up and remains vital for health and growth. While every child needs a daily dose of active play, the physical benefits are invaluable for children with stiff and sore joints. Active play helps maintain energy and increases joint flexibility as well as muscle strength. You cannot reasonably expect a young child to take part in repetitive exercises, but you can usually get him or her to play.

With some creativity and a little ingenuity, it is possible to persuade every child with arthritis to be actively engaged in play. Your child needs to be careful with exercise choices. For instance, it is best to

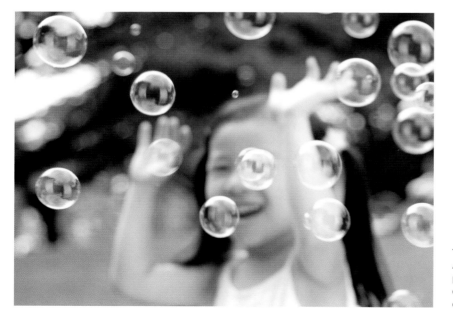

THE IMPORTANCE OF PLAY
Active play that avoids overuse of particularly hot or inflamed joints is essential to the health and growth of every child with arthritis.

Joining a support group can provide the family with help, advice, and guidance as well as the chance to talk to other young people and parents of children with arthritis.

avoid contact sports and activities that will overuse one part of the body. It is also important to avoid activities that stress those joints that are hot or inflamed. However, it is also essential to encourage activities that keep children with their friends.

Special needs at home

Without question, arthritis in children imposes physical and psychological stresses on family life. Even the most stable of families struggle to establish and maintain a sensible balance in the order of things. When the child needs special care, the strain on keeping that balance is increased exponentially. Family relationships may suffer when parents set aside too much time for the child.

When the arthritis is particularly bad, the child feels too unwell to take part in any activity, causing complex problems within the family. Try to make adjustments and contingency plans. The family needs to accept such uncertainties with equanimity, and to encourage ideas for activities on active days and quiet days.

Family members should try to help by treating the child with arthritis as normally as possible, while ensuring that he or she receives suitable medical care. Vitally important, too, is the need to explain to the child that getting arthritis is no one's fault. Occasionally, children believe that their arthritis is a repayment for something they did.

Joining a support group can provide the family with help, advice, and guidance as well as the chance to talk to other young people and parents of children with arthritis.

Long-term outlook

Overall, the prognosis for juvenile arthritis is relatively good. With modern techniques of treatment and management, most children do well.

The long-term outlook for pauciarticular juvenile arthritis is very good. However, this is not true of polyarthritis because there is a substantial risk of progressive and destructive arthritis as well as joint deformities. This is especially true if rheumatoid factor is present (see p.41).

The long-term outlook of systemic arthritis depends on the organs affected and if it progresses to polyarticular disease.

Complications can be very worrisome in a small number of

TALK TO YOUR CHILD
Spending time talking to a child with arthritis will help him or her understand the nature of the illness and will bring you closer as a family.

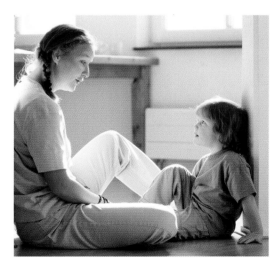

children. Complications, such as infection, inflammation of the heart, and kidney disease, can prematurely claim the lives of between 1 and 5 percent of children with juvenile arthritis.

The effect on growth

Many children with juvenile chronic arthritis, especially those with systemic or polyarthritis, do not grow normally. One typical feature is a small lower jaw and a small chin.

Chronic inflammation and steroid treatment are the main causes, with contributions from poor nutrition due to decreased appetite as well as limited physical activity. However, active treatment and the careful use of minimal doses of steroids can reduce the degree of retarded growth.

The longer juvenile arthritis continues, the more likely the inflamed joints and surrounding muscles and tendons will become damaged. What effect prolonged inflammation has depends on which joints are most involved.

Typical problems include the inability to bend and straighten the knees properly, shortened legs, and damage to the small joints of the hand. Sometimes, the joints in the neck are damaged.

However, orthopedic surgeons can replace joints that fail (see p.92), release joints that cannot straighten properly, and remove damaged cartilage from a joint.

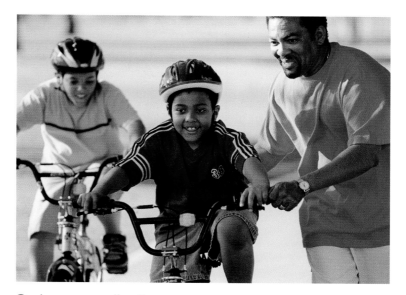

Serious complications

Some children with arthritis can develop serious organ problems, due either to the disease or its treatment with drugs. Problems include an inflamed pericardium (the membrane around the heart) and kidney failure. Inflammation of the blood vessels (see p.34) can affect many different organs.

Uveitis, in which the uvea layer of the eye becomes inflamed, is potentially debilitating and can result in blindness. Expert care and monitoring from eye surgeons can minimize the risks.

Children who have prolonged and widespread inflammation that is left untreated can accumulate a protein called amyloid throughout the body. This causes failure of individual organs, such as the kidneys. However, with modern treatments this complication is becoming increasingly rare.

ENCOURAGING GROWTH
Physical activity, along with good nutrition and careful use of steroids, can encourage growth and minimize the chances of retarded growth.

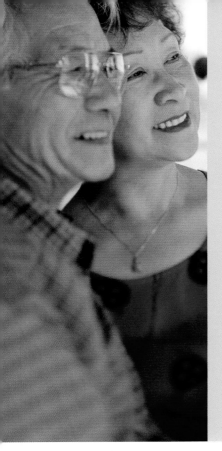

People at special risk

Some people are more prone than others to developing one of the many forms of arthritis. Women represent the largest group because they experience menopause, a time of hormonal change that is associated with an increased incidence of arthritis and osteoporosis. Other special risk groups include people who put their joints under persistent or repetitive strain—athletes, manual workers, and obese individuals—and people who are genetically predisposed to arthritis.

HT not only helps increase the density of bone but may also prevent osteoarthritis of the knee.

Postmenopause and arthritis

Arthritis affects more women in the general population than men. But age is an important factor in this picture; the biggest proportion of women with arthritis are post-menopausal. This is the time in a woman's life when she is most likely to suffer from osteoarthritis or rheumatoid arthritis. As if this susceptibility was not enough, a postmenopausal woman is at an increased risk of developing osteoporosis, as well.

After menopause a woman's body changes in many different ways because her ovaries have stopped producing the hormones estrogen and progesterone. Among the many apparent results of this hormonal change is an increased risk of developing osteoarthritis, particularly of the knees and hands. As a result, osteoarthritis is much more common in women of this age (late 40s to early 50s) than in men of the same age.

The link between estrogen and osteoarthritis is still not completely understood, but many studies seem to suggest that a link does exist. Australian researchers, for example, have found that hormone replacement therapy (HT) not only

Q&A

If I take corticosteroids, what is the risk that I will develop osteoporosis?

Anyone who takes corticosteroids for more than 3 months has an increased risk of developing osteoporosis, and the risk increases if you:

● Have a family history of the disease.

● Have had previous fractures.

● Have ever had anorexia nervosa.

● Smoke or abuse alcohol.

● Take certain medications, such as the blood thinner heparin.

helps increase the density of bone but may also prevent osteoarthritis of the knee.

Doctors in the US found that when women are receiving treatments for conditions that deplete the estrogen in the body, as with some breast cancer drugs, they are more prone to developing joint pain and swelling. However, it is unlikely to be recommended by doctors as a treatment for osteoarthritis alone because of the possible risks associated with taking HT (see p.195).

Osteoporosis

Osteoporosis, which literally means "porous bone," is a disease that causes the bones in the body to become less dense and more fragile (see p.35). In women, the hormone estrogen plays an important role in keeping bones

strong, so the loss of estrogen after menopause significantly increases the loss of bone density and consequently the risk of osteoporosis.

One in three women over the age of 50 will suffer a fracture. Women who have had an early menopause, a hysterectomy (removal of the uterus), or their ovaries removed before the age of 45 are also at risk of developing osteoporosis.

Rheumatoid arthritis and osteoporosis

Women are two to three times more likely to develop rheumatoid arthritis than men. At the same time, if you have rheumatoid arthritis you are also more likely to develop osteoporosis.

There may be several reasons for this link. First, the inflammation and pain of rheumatoid arthritis

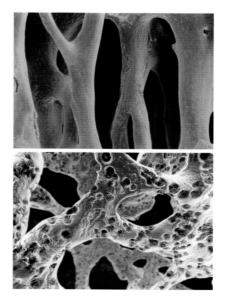

HEALTHY BONE
Normal spongy bone (left) contains trabeculae, which are like struts that are both light and strong. Bone marrow fills the space in between the trabeculae.

OSTEOPOROSIS
In osteoporosis (left), the fabric of the spongy bone tissue becomes less dense and more brittle. Here, a vertebra affected by osteoporosis shows the typical porosity, visible as small dark areas in the bone.

may prevent or deter women from regular exercise, which can also have a negative effect on the strength of their bones.

Second, studies show that rheumatoid arthritis can make you more susceptible to osteoporosis because of the bone loss that may occur around affected joints.

SOURCES OF CALCIUM

The average recommended daily amount (RDA) by the government is currently 700mg of calcium for men and women, but if you already have osteoporosis you may need up to 1200mg. The chart below provides some guidelines on how much calcium is present in certain foods.

FOOD	WEIGHT	CALCIUM CONTENT
Whole milk	1/3 pint (190ml)	224mg
Low-fat milk	1/3 pint (190ml)	231mg
Skim milk	1/3 pint (190ml)	235mg
Low-fat yogurt	5oz (150g)	225mg
Ice cream	4oz (112g)	134 mg
Cheddar cheese	1oz (28g)	202mg
Boiled spinach	4oz (112g)	179mg
Baked beans	4oz (112g)	59mg
White bread (1 slice)	1oz (28g)	33mg
1 large orange		58mg
Dried apricots	3 1/2 oz (100g)	92mg
Brazil nuts	3 1/2 oz (100g)	170mg
Sardines (canned)	3 oz (84g)	325mg
Salmon (canned)	2 oz (56g)	52mg

Finally, if you take corticosteroids for the pain and inflammation of rheumatoid arthritis, there is a significant risk that you will have some reduction in bone density.

Preventing osteoporosis

The best way of preventing osteoporosis, or at least slowing its progress, is to take enough calcium and vitamins, especially vitamin D, and to engage in regular weight-bearing exercise. Your doctor may prescribe drugs called bisphosphonates or SERMs, which are bone-protecting agents.

Calcium

This mineral is vital for the health of your bones. Good sources of calcium (see left) include foods such as dairy products. You don't need whole versions because low-and non-fat dairy products contain as much and sometimes even more calcium as the fattier versions.

You also find calcium in Brazil nuts, dried beans, dark-green leafy vegetables such as spinach, kale and broccoli, as well as in canned salmon and sardines that contain the bones. Some foods such as bread and orange juice are fortified with extra calcium.

If you don't think you can include enough calcium in your diet, add a little powdered milk to some recipes, such as desserts or soups, or ask your doctor about taking a supplement.

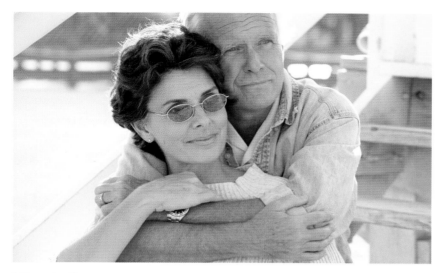

GET SOME SUN
Regular sunlight helps you produce vitamin D, which in turn helps you absorb calcium.

Vitamin D

This vitamin plays an important part in helping absorb calcium. If you spend time in the sun without a sunscreen on a regular basis you will make all the vitamin D you need. Dietary sources include egg yolks, some vitamin-enriched foods, and supplements. Limited evidence suggests that vitamin D may help in osteoarthritis, too.

Exercise

Regular exercise builds up the strength of your bones and muscles. Weight-bearing exercise is the best type because it forces you to work against gravity and helps minimize loss of minerals, such as calcium, from the bones. Walking, climbing stairs, and dancing are all good examples of beneficial weight-bearing exercise.

However, if you already have developed osteoporosis, walking for half an hour a day is the best form of exercise because it puts the least stress on your bones. You may be reluctant to exercise if you have arthritis, but it is vital that joints are given enough movement to prevent further damage and pain (see pp.64–71 and pp.158–171). You should also ask your physician about your weight.

Hormone therapy

Hormone therapy, or HT, is the term given to drugs containing estrogen and progesterone, which are no longer produced by the body during and after menopause.

Many women, regardless of whether or not they already have arthritis, experience a range of bothersome or unpleasant symptoms both before and after menopause. These symptoms include hot flashes, dry skin, irritability, and depression. Some women also experience

REGULAR EXERCISE
Exercising regularly is a crucial part of maintaining the health of your bones and preventing osteoporosis.

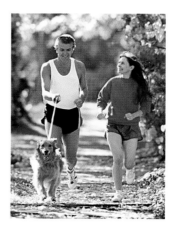

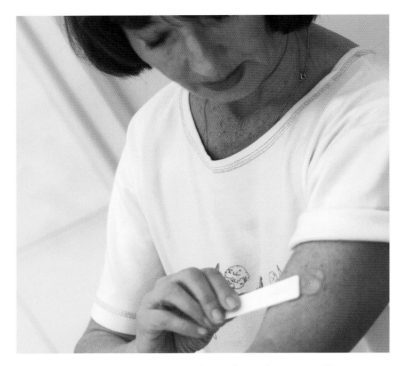

HRT PATCH
Adhesive patches are a simple and effective way of delivering HT drugs slowly and directly into the bloodstream.

The perceived wisdom on HT had been that it actually protected women from heart disease and strokes.

a loss of sex drive as well as discomfort during sex.

HT is the standard treatment for these symptoms. It is taken in the form of pills, patches worn on the skin, implants placed just under the skin, or vaginal pills, creams, or membranes.

Women who have undergone menopause early, or have had a hysterectomy or their ovaries removed at an early age, are often offered HT. Women who have not had a hysterectomy will usually take a combination of estrogen and a progestational agent. Those who have had a hysterectomy use estrogen-only preparations

HT has been shown to protect against osteoporosis. It is also possible that this therapy may

offer some protection against osteoarthritis in postmenopausal women.

The risks of HT

Taking HT has been associated with several serious health risks, including breast cancer, blood clots, and cardiovascular disease.

■ **BREAST CANCER** If HT is taken for less than 5 years there doesn't appear to be any increased risk of breast cancer, but after this time there is a small increase. A major study, known as the Million Women Study, appeared to show the biggest risk of breast cancer is posed by HT when it combines estrogen and progesterone.

When a woman has not had a hysterectomy, progesterone protects against endometrial cancer, so doctors will still advise her to take the combined hormones. Taking HT does not appear to increase the risk of breast cancer further when women take it at a younger age than the norm—for example, after a premature menopause or an early hysterectomy. The 5-year risk period seems to begin from the age of 50. After 5 years, for all women, the risk appears to revert back to the normal rate.

■ **BLOOD CLOTS** Taking HT appears to carry a slightly higher than normal risk of developing a blood clot, or venous thromboembolism (VTE). If you are already in a risk group for VTE, you should not take HT.

■ **CARDIOVASCULAR DISEASE** In the past, it was felt that HT protected women from heart disease and strokes. Most experts now believe there is no protection from HT. The Food and Drug Administration believes that, in the long term, the risks of HT outweigh its benefits.

Is HT worth the risk?

In the US the consensus seems to be that for women who experience the more distressing symptoms of menopause or early menopause, the benefits of HT usually outweigh the risks for short-term use at the lowest dose.

HT is not recommended as a drug therapy for the treatment of osteoporosis alone. As with any form of medication, both prescription and over-the-counter, it is important that you talk to your physician about your particular circumstances and whether the drug in question is right for you.

Sporting risks

Super-fit people, such as professional athletes, who constantly train and play a particular sport, regularly have an increased risk of arthritis. This is because any trauma on a joint—whether from persistent repetitive movement, overuse, or a sports injury—can make the joint more susceptible to developing arthritis.

Depending on which joint is overused, the severity of the trauma, and the intensity of the inflammation that is produced

PLAYING SOCCER
The sudden twists, turns, and tackles in a game of soccer can expose players to joint damage that could lead to arthritis later.

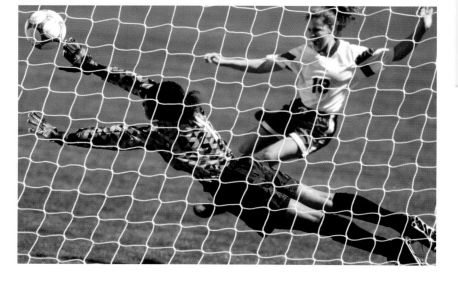

as a result of the damage to cartilage and soft tissues, a degree of osteoarthritis is likely.

Repetitive trauma carries a high risk of future problems. One example is osteoarthritis of the knee (see p.17) in former soccer players, many of whom will need knee replacement surgery (see p.94) at a relatively early age.

Occupational risks

Occupations involving repetitive knee bending or an increased risk of injury to the knee joints, particularly a repetitive injury, are associated with the development of osteoarthritis later in life. Examples include heavy manual labor in industries such as construction and agriculture. Less physically taxing professions are also affected. Dancers and musicians are particularly prone to overuse of their joints—for example, the bowing shoulder of violinists and the hands of pianists are commonly affected. Other joints that may be affected by overuse and repetitive injuries include hips, wrists, shoulders, and lower back (see pp.28–31).

MECHANICAL VIBRATION
Drills, jack hammers, and other sources of mechnical vibration can cause carpal tunnel syndrome and repetitive strain injury.

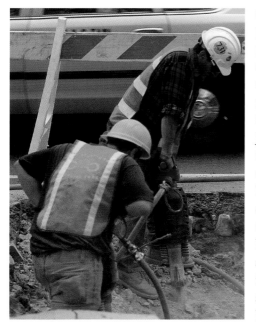

Obesity

People who are obese are at much greater risk of developing knee osteoarthritis than people who are a healthy weight for their height. This is especially so for women. Obesity is usually defined as having a body mass index (BMI) of 30 or more. You can calculate your BMI by measuring your height in inches and weight in pounds (see opposite). Studies have shown that for every increase in BMI above 27, the risk of developing knee osteoarthritis increases by 15 percent. Losing weight may help reduce this risk (see p.62).

Being overweight or obese can lead to osteoarthritis in several ways. First, being overweight increases the amount of force on weight-bearing joints, such as the knees. Second, the fatty tissues may alter the person's balance of hormones, which could affect cartilage and bone tissues. Third, obese people have relatively weak muscles, are less fit than normal, and injure themselves more often.

Ethnic groups

The relationship between ethnicity and arthritis is complex. From a genetic point of view, a particular ethnic group may be predisposed or more prone to a particular type of arthritis. Added to this is the fact that different groups receive—for

CALCULATING BODY MASS INDEX (BMI)

Body mass index (BMI) is the relationship of your weight to your height, and is calculated by dividing your weight in pounds by the square of your height in inches, and multiplied by 703. For example, a man who weighs 220lb and is 71in tall has a BMI of 30.68. The chart below will help place your BMI in one of four groups, from underweight to obese.

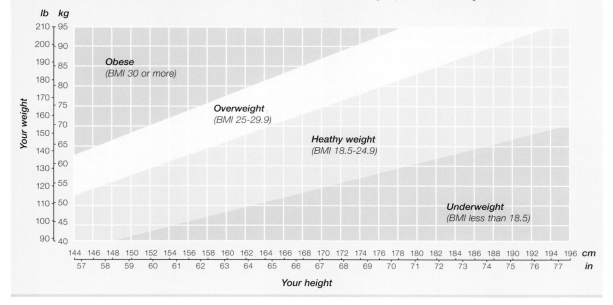

whatever reason—different levels of medical care, which affects the way their arthritis is treated.

Finally, members of different ethnic groups respond in different ways to apparently similar clinical problems. For example, the way individuals respond to pain and disability is very dependent on their overall view of the world and the support they receive from their family and community.

Ethnicity and rheumatoid arthritis

Variations in the frequency of rheumatoid arthritis have been studied in different ethnic groups.

In most Western countries, the disease affects an average of about 1 percent of adults (1.5 percent of women and 0.6 percent of men). Lower rates have been reported in China, Japan, parts of Greece, and rural Africa. It seems particularly uncommon in West Africa.

Conversely, there appears to be a high prevalence in several Native American populations, such as the Tlingit of Southeast Alaska, the Yakima of central Washington, and the Pima of Arizona. The high rate of rheumatoid arthritis in these populations leads to speculation about their unique genetic or environmental factors. The clinical

From a genetic point of view, a particular ethnic group may be predisposed or more prone to a particular type of arthritis.

For many years, rheumatologists have known that genetics play a strong role in ankylosing spondylitis.

features of rheumatoid arthritis in these Native Americans are different from those of the normal population: the disease is more severe, often starts at a younger age, and a family history is more common. This prevalence and severity strongly suggests that genetics play an important role.

Ethnicity and osteoarthritis

Some forms of osteoarthritis, such as generalized osteoarthritis that involves the hand, are found predominantly in Caucasians. Conversely, good evidence indicates that hand and foot osteoarthritis is uncommon in Africans. However, the situation is complex because knee osteoarthritis is common in African Americans. Finally, some groups have very low rates of osteoarthritis of the hip, including Chinese and Japanese populations.

Inherited markers or traits

The inherited nature of arthritis has been known for many years, mainly from family studies that show that if one member of a family has rheumatoid arthritis or ankylosing spondylitis it is more likely to be found in other family members. Studies of twins lend even more support to this inheritance: when one has the disease the other is more likely to have it if the twins are identical

than fraternal. Nevertheless, both twins have rheumatoid arthritis in less than 50% of cases.

Studying the genetics of people with arthritis suggests that there are marker genes or traits in their chromosomes, especially the HLA–DR4 marker in rheumatoid arthritis and the HLA–B27 marker in ankylosing spondylitis.

HLA–DR4 in rheumatoid arthritis

Genetic studies in rheumatoid arthritis have concentrated on white blood cells, especially the major histocompatibility complex (MHC) group of genes.

Scientists have discovered that one of these genes, known as HLA–DR4, is present in some people with rheumatoid arthritis but not others. They think that there is a link between this discovery and the geographical variation of rheumatoid arthritis.

Q&A

Both my father and my mother suffered from arthritis—does this mean that I will develop it, too?

Not necessarily. According to research, some forms of arthritis may well be linked to certain genes and may therefore be inherited. But this is not inevitable. There do seem to be other triggers such as infections that can bring on arthritis. Besides, rheumatologists are uncertain about the causes of many types of arthritis.

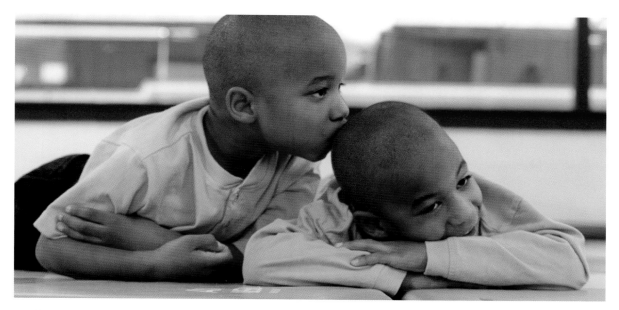

Evidence suggests that people who have the HLA–DR4 gene have rheumatoid arthritis more severely and are more likely to have rheumatoid nodules and erosion of the bones within their joints.

Since the gene is important in determining how the immune system works, scientists thought they were on the verge of a breakthrough. To date, they have been unable to unravel the story further. As a result, the knowledge that someone has the HLA-DR4 gene has not yet influenced the treatment of rheumatoid arthritis.

HLA–B27 in ankylosing spondylitis

For many years, rheumatologists have known that genetics play a strong role in ankylosing spondylitis. In the early 1970s, scientists showed that this was due to the presence of a gene known as HLA–B27, which also belongs to the MHC group.

About 95 percent of people with ankylosing spondylitis have this genetic marker, compared to 8 percent of the general population. HLA–B27 is also found, but with less frequency, in other conditions that are associated with ankylosing spondylitis. These include uveitis (eye inflammation) and psoriatic arthritis (see p.22).

One or more environmental triggers lead to ankylosing spondylitis in a minority (about 5–10 percent) of people who have the HLA–27 gene. Many of these triggers are likely to be infections, particularly infections in the bowel or pelvis. Those populations with a high rate of rheumatoid arthritis, such as the Pima of Arizona, often have HLA-B27, too.

IDENTICAL TWINS
The genes of identical twins reveal that when one twin develops arthritis the other one is more likely to develop it, too.

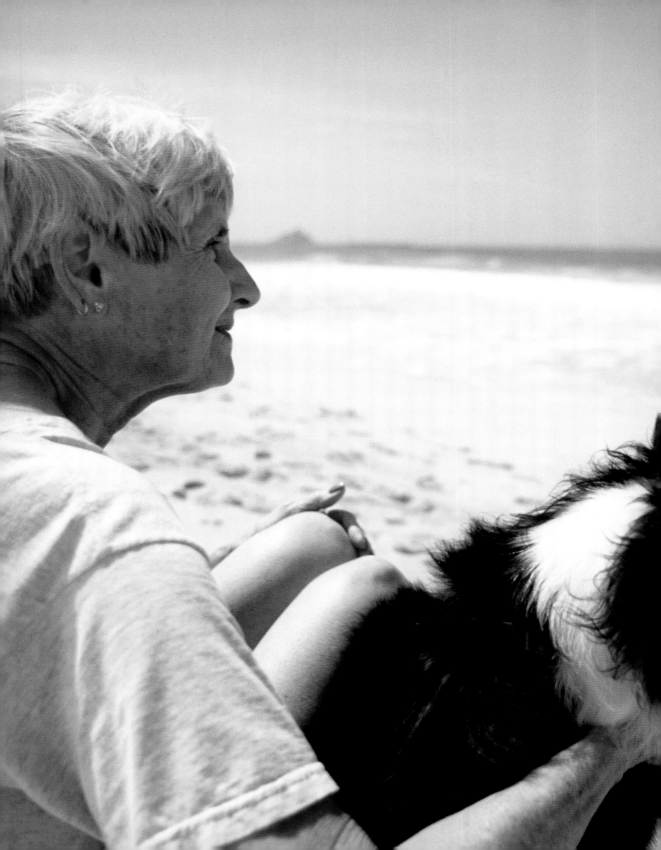

Long-term outlook

The management and treatment of arthritis has improved greatly over the years but there has been no cure. This gradual progress is probably the most realistic scenario for the future, too—rather than expecting breakthroughs that lead to a cure, it seems more rational to think in terms of continuing small improvements.

Perhaps the true aim of treating arthritis is to ensure that everyone with arthritis can achieve a good response to treatment while keeping disability to a minimum.

Progress in managing arthritis comes with increased prevention, early intervention, and better treatments. In the past it has also come with a significant increase in the number of arthritis specialists, in the improved access to a range of healthcare professionals, and in the development of many new treatments.

However, most forms of arthritis increase with age—as people continue to live longer they are likely to have more arthritis rather than less. The demographic time bomb underlying the aging of western populations is likely to increase the chronic diseases of later life, including arthritis.

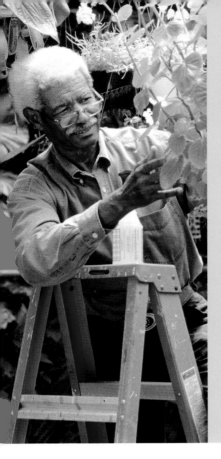

The outlook for arthritis

As with many long-term conditions, the outlook for anyone with arthritis is hard to predict. From year to year, changes may affect your prognosis—some for the better, such as a new treatment or a spontaneous improvement in your symptoms. On the other hand, life with arthritis can get more complicated if new health problems arise or when aging starts to make itself felt. However, one thing is certain. Taking an active part in your own health care will give you the best chance of managing your arthritis well.

Mild osteoarthritis does not necessarily become worse and could remain relatively stable for the rest of your life.

What's likely to happen?

Most people with arthritis can expect to lead full lives, enjoying as many years as anyone else for following a career, participating in leisure activities, and having relationships. If you are newly diagnosed, you will need time to make adjustments both physically and mentally but, with the help of healthcare specialists, you will learn more about your condition and find the confidence to cope.

What happens in the years after your diagnosis depends on the management of your condition, on the type of arthritis you have, and how it affects you as an individual. Although many forms of arthritis have a broad recognizable pattern, no physician will be able to tell you with absolute certainty what your personal prognosis might be.

Osteoarthritis
Mild osteoarthritis (see p.14) does not necessarily become worse and could remain relatively stable for the rest of your life. In later years, you may have no greater problems with mobility than would be normal with aging. You may find that your symptoms tend to vary: for example, pain and stiffness may ease in warmer weather.

Rheumatoid arthritis

The pattern for most people with rheumatoid arthritis (see p.18) is for symptoms flare up for a period, then die down or disappear for weeks or even months. The amount of damage to the joints depends on how severe flare-ups are and how often they occur. Eventually, you may have some degree of permanent stiffness. However, you will probably be able to continue with your normal life, since severe disability is uncommon. Very rarely, flare-ups can cease altogether; but if this does happen, any joint damage is likely to remain permanent.

Ankylosing spondylitis

The outlook for most people with ankylosing spondylitis (see p.21) is good. Severe disability is not usual because treatment (especially regular exercise or physical

Q&A

Does rheumatoid arthritis put me at greater risk of developing other diseases in the long term?

Possibly. Studies suggest conditions such as heart disease, osteoporosis stroke, and infections may be more likely. One reason may be that people with rheumatoid arthritis are not able to exercise freely. In some cases, the drugs for rheumatoid arthritis can raise blood pressure (a risk factor for stroke) or inhibit the immune system, making infections more likely.

therapy) is very effective in preventing joint stiffness. If you have the condition, you have a reasonable chance of being only mildly affected in your daily life.

Changes in long-term treatment

You may be taking a drug that suits you and has kept your symptoms well controlled for many years. But sometimes, for reasons not related to arthritis, this drug may stop being an option. From midlife onward, other health problems start to become more common. In some cases, they are made worse by your arthritis drugs or require medication that interacts with your existing arthritis treatment.

For example, if you develop high blood pressure you may not be able to take steroids to reduce inflammation, because they raise blood pressure. Anticlotting drugs for a cardiovascular disorder cannot be taken with certain types of NSAID, which also have an anticlotting effect. If you develop a kidney or liver disease, you will not be able to take some disease-modifying antirheumatic drugs (see p.83) because their potential side effects include damage to the kidneys or liver.

If you do need to discontinue an arthritis drug or to take a mixture of drugs for different conditions, your doctor will advise you on the

PRACTICAL TIPS

REDUCING THE RISK OF LONG-TERM PROBLEMS

● Take an active part in managing your arthritis.

● Stay as physically active as possible. Maintain your mobility and exercise your joints and muscles regularly.

● Eat a well-balanced diet.

● Keep your weight to a healthy level (see p.199).

● Don't smoke or drink excessively.

● Follow your physician's instructions and keep taking your medication

● Make sure you are tested and monitored regularly so that problems can be spotted—and treated—sooner rather than later.

Improved materials and surgical procedures mean that implants now work better for longer than they did in the past.

REGULAR EXERCISE
The importance of regular exercise cannot be emphasized enough—just resist the temptation to overdo it by going beyond reasonable limits.

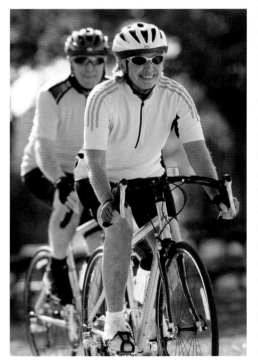

best course of action. In some cases, you may need to take medication for a possibly life-threatening disease at the expense of controlling your arthritis. It is all a question of balance.

Keeping a replacement joint working

Joint replacement surgery can be life-changing, giving back mobility to people who thought they would never enjoy normal activities again. As a result of improved materials and surgical procedures, implants now work better for longer than they did in the past. Your implant could serve you well for up to 20 years—but it won't last forever. So what can you expect in the long term?

Inevitably, with wear and tear, replacement joints tend to loosen over time, becoming less efficient or causing pain. If this happens, it may be necessary to perform revision surgery (see p.107) to prevent damage within the joint and possible further disability. Surgery the second time round takes longer and is

more complicated than the initial operation. Recovery is likely to take longer, too.

You can do a lot to get the best from a replacement joint and to protect it from early deterioration. Get regular exercise to keep the implant mobile, but don't be tempted to go beyond reasonable limits, however fit you feel. In particular, avoid high-impact activities or sudden movements that subject the joint to excessive stresses and strains. A fall can seriously damage an implant, so take precautions by making sure your home is safe and free from hazards that are easy to trip over.

Problems in the elderly

Although arthritis is not just a condition that occurs in later life, some forms—particularly osteoarthritis and rheumatoid arthritis—are far more likely to develop in older people. By the time they reach their 50s or 60s, over 30 percent of people have some symptoms of arthritis.

The frequency of arthritis rises with increasing age: some 60 percent of those over 85 years old are affected. Because people are living longer—at least, in the developed world—they are more and more often having to deal with the challenges that arise when their arthritis combines with the unique problems of old age.

Reduced movement

The elderly have weaker muscles than younger people, so they find it more difficult to cope with the way arthritis affects their mobility. It is harder for them to stay active enough to maintain strength and fitness through exercise, so their disability is likely to increase. Their movement can be further restricted by joint or bone damage not related to arthritis, such as a fracture of the hip or shoulder caused by a fall. However, in many instances, simple measures such as a program of supervised walking can make an important difference.

Coping with drug treatment

Drugs for treating arthritis tend to have a more toxic effect in elderly people. This is partly because the older we get the less efficient our bodies become at breaking down drugs. Also, older people are more likely to be taking drugs for other conditions and these may interact with arthritis drugs (see p.205). For this reason, physicians keep the dosages to a minimum and carefully monitor their older patients to watch for reactions.

Living with arthritis

Arthritis won't just go away—but that doesn't mean you have to regard the condition as a life sentence of increasing disability and pain. For one thing, with specialist support available, you have expert help in keeping your

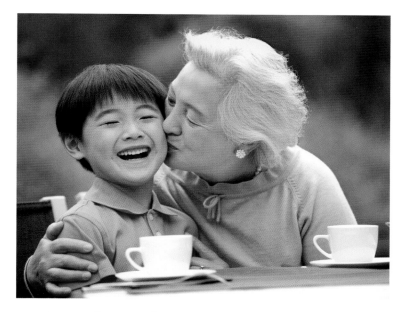

symptoms under control. Physicians, therapists, nurses, and researchers work as a team to make your arthritis as managable as possible. One of the most important team members is you.

There is a lot that only you can do to improve your outlook. Even the most highly effective drugs will not work unless you are committed to following the instructions of your physician and to taking your medication regularly.

Many aspects of general health that make a big difference to your arthritis are under your control too. For example, you can choose whether or not to exercise to improve strength and mobility, to eat sensibly, to maintain a healthy weight, or to avoid damaging your body by smoking or excess drinking. Good self-management is an essential part of your treatment.

ENJOYING PLEASURE
People with arthritis have every reason to enjoy the pleasures of laughter, fun, and happiness.

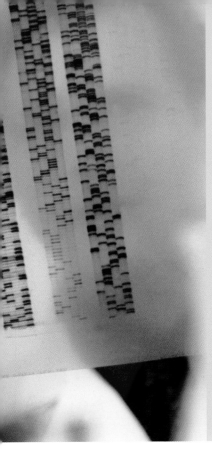

Arthritis in the future

As with many other conditions, scientists are working to find a cure for arthritis. However, no one expects the discovery of a wonder drug that will cure all symptoms in everyone. But as research progresses, understanding of arthritis in all its diverse forms continues to increase, thereby increasing the possibility of improvements in the management and treatment of the disease. Ongoing clinical trials are testing powerful new medications and therapies that have the potential to significantly reduce the disabilities caused by arthritis.

Medical researchers are trying to develop appropriate medications in various potential avenues, and are trying to make significant breakthroughs.

Making progress

Without doubt, considerable progress in treating the various forms of arthritis has been made over the years. Not least, there has been great improvements in three important areas: better surgical techniques to replace joints, an increase in the number of arthritis specialists, and improved access to a range of specialized expertise and healthcare professionals.

Broad lines of research

It is difficult to speculate about the future of arthritis and arthritis care, but there are several broad lines of research. In the simplest approach, clinicians look at ways of maximizing the effectiveness of current treatments, focusing particularly on the timing of drug therapy and how different drugs can be combined.

In another approach, various pharmaceutical companies are working to develop innovative treatments, either by making small improvements to tried and tested drugs or by introducing entirely new ones.

Other avenues of research include studies on the role of genetics in arthritis and the link between infection and joint inflammation.

The development of new drugs

Since arthritis is a common and long-lasting disease, and it is widespread among all populations and age groups, it is a natural target for research into new drugs.

The pharmaceutical industry will continue to research and deliver new drugs and medications to treat the various forms of arthritis. From a commercial point of view, the financial rewards for success would be substantial because the market is so large.

Developing successful new drugs takes pharmaceutical companies many years of painstaking research and is enormously expensive. Most of the drugs they investigate fail to make the grade because their benefits are limited or they have an excessively toxic effect.

However, every decade sees the development of new drugs, each with some unique benefits over their predecessors. Not all of these drugs stand the test of time, but most do.

Drug prospects

Trials to test the effectiveness of drugs (see p.213) are valuable because they can focus on the causes of arthritis or of its ultimate effects on joint damage. Medical researchers are trying to develop appropriate medications in various potential avenues, and are trying to make significant breakthroughs.

■ **ANTIBIOTICS** If pharmaceutical research showed that a type of arthritis was caused by infection, drug companies would try to develop a specific antibiotic to prevent it.

■ **DISEASE-MODIFYING DRUG** A drug that effectively blocks, or inhibits, the enzymes involved in joint damage could have the potential to be a disease-modifying drug in the treatment of osteoarthritis.

■ **ORAL TNF–ALPHA BLOCKERS** Another prospect on the horizon is the development of second generation TNF–alpha blockers (see p.85), which can be taken by mouth. The first generation of these relatively new drugs have to be administered

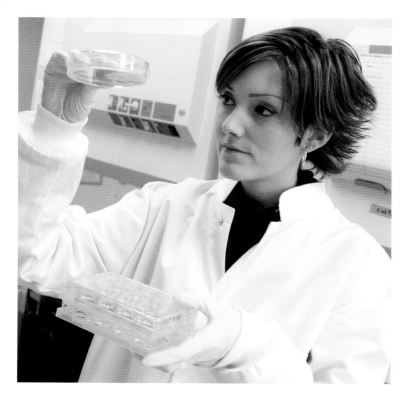

MEDICAL RESEARCH
Many years of careful medical research are required before a potential drug is fully tested and available for prescription.

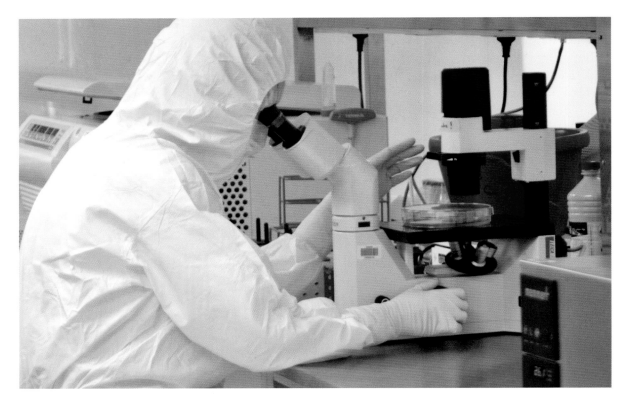

MICROSCOPIC EXAMINATION
Medical research, even looking through a microscpe at the effects of a drug on biological tissue, is conducted in hygienic conditions.

by injection, although many people with rheumatoid arthritis are happy to accept injections as necessary if their disease can remain better controlled.

■ **IMPROVED ANALGESICS** A need that has not yet been met to any great extent is for improved analgesics. There have been many attempts, but almost all have fallen by the wayside for one reason or another. To discover a safe and effective analgesic that causes few side effects may be impossible.

■ **REVERSING JOINT DAMAGE** The ultimate goal is to design a drug that will reduce or even reverse joint damage in all types of arthritis. Several potential drugs

have been tried in research studies and although none has yet proved successful there is a good chance that an ideal drug will eventually be identified.

Testing biologic agents
The most likely area for new drug developments lies in identifying biologic agents (see p.85) that can block, or inhibit, one or more of the pathways in inflammation.

This is a challenging task, since there are a host of different targets in the body, such as the small chemicals called cytokines, that might be relevant. Some 30 or so biologic agents are being tested at present, of which at least a quarter, perhaps more, will become available for treating inflammatory arthritis over the next couple of decades.

This work raises the possibility of discovering more specific biologic agents to target the rarer diseases, such as ankylosing spondylitis, psoriatic arthritis, reactive arthritis, and lupus.

Eventually, medical research may even lead to the evolution of a combination therapy (see p.87) in which several biologic agents— each affecting a different cytokine —suppress or even cure rheumatoid arthritis.

Investigating infections

Doctors are learning more about the link between infections and arthritis. In some people, infection causes a fault in the immune system so that substances produced by the body to fight the infection also attack the tissue of healthy joints—and scientists are trying to find out exactly why.

Their experiments have shown that it may be possible to block the damaging effects of a faulty immune system without affecting its protective mechanism. This avenue of research could have exciting implications, both for identifying people at risk of developing arthritis and for the prevention and treatment of arthritis in the future.

Stem cell transplants

A pioneering procedure causing much interest and excitement is stem cell transplantation, which has been used successfully to treat a few extreme cases of arthritis. Stem cells are immature cells, formed in bone marrow, that have the potential to develop into more specialized cells, such as those that play a part in the immune system.

In transplantation, the stem cells are taken from a person's blood, then purified and stored. In the next step, the person's immune cells are destroyed with drugs and the stem cells are put back into the blood. If all goes well, these stem cells will develop into healthy immune cells.

In rheumatoid arthritis, a disease caused by a faulty immune system,

STEM CELLS
Depending on the biochemical signal that it receives, each of the stem cells in this clump has the potential to grow and develop into any type of cell in the body.

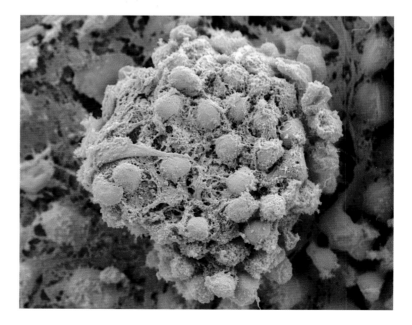

stem cell transplantation can have a dramatic effect and symptoms may be greatly reduced or even disappear altogether.

The treatment has potential for future development. Researchers are also experimenting with the possibility of using stem cell transplants to repair cartilage damaged by osteoarthritis.

Risks of stem cell transplants

The procedure of transplanting stem cells is extremely risky because it leaves the individual temporarily without any immune system at all. As a result, he or she is highly vulnerable to even the most minor infections. and has to remain isolated in the hospital until the new immune system is firmly established. There is also the possibility that the stem cells themselves will become faulty.

For these reasons, stem cell transplantation has been used only as a last option when every other treatment for severe arthritis has been ineffective.

The genetic approach

The study of genes and the practice of gene therapy is often heralded as the future direction of research into rheumatic diseases and the opening of a door to a new age of treatment.

The theory is that the analysis of an individual's genes will reveal the biological factors that drive his or her arthritis. At the same time, it will allow an evaluation of the person's potential responses to specific drugs, whether they are disease-modifiers or biologic agents. Equipped with this unique, individualized information, medical researchers and healthcare professionals would be able to devise a tailor-made treatment.

However, this approach has so far borne little fruit. The expense of analyzing a person's genes and developing a drug regime that will probably only benefit them is not attractive proposition for a pharmaceutical company used to making sizeable profits. Yet this individualized treatment is almost certain to happen one day, but no one knows when it will become routine. It is most likely to benefit us in the distant future.

GENOME RESEARCH
A fully automated gene production line uses a robot and a computer vision system to select and deliver particular sequences of DNA that enable scientists to investigate an individual's genes.

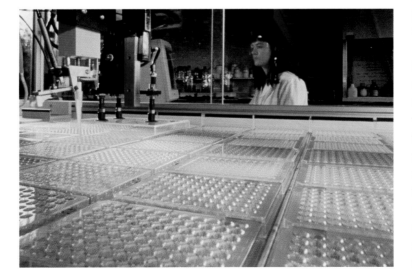

Improvements in surgery

Techniques and materials for joint replacement surgery continue to improve and the effectiveness of treatment is constantly being evaluated. In one line of research, medical scientists are investigating the reasons why artificial joints fail in certain people after a relatively short time. They are endeavoring to identify biological markers that could predict which individuals are more likely to be susceptible to infection or to the premature loosening of an implant.

Researchers are also examining ways of developing better types of cement for joint replacements in the knee and hip. In addition, advances in imaging techniques to study joints may result in better designs for implants as well as more efficient surgery.

Q&A

If I take part in trials of a new drug, does this mean I can get the latest treatment and what are the risks?

Taking part in a clinical trial does not guarantee access to state-of-the-art drugs. Some participants are given a placebo drug—that is, a tablet that contains no medication and therefore has no effect. Drug trials can never be entirely free of risk because the new medications, although already subjected to rigorous tests, may have side effects that have not previously come to light.

How you can help with research

If you have arthritis there are ways you can contribute to research. Doctors and scientists need your personal experience to help them build up databanks of information.

Thousands of people volunteer to participate in clinical trials, in which new or revised treatments are tested on people by monitoring their effectiveness and long-term safety.

These carefully controlled trials require a degree of commitment because they can extend for two or three years or longer. For the duration of the trial, you may have to discontinue taking any drugs that you are currently prescribed, possibly making your arthritis less well controlled than it is now. If you feel you may be a suitable candidate for a drug trial, ask your physician or specialist for information and advice.

Participating in surveys

You can help medical researchers by taking part in surveys to collect data from people with arthritis on such issues as pain, disability, side-effects of medication, and lifestyle. Your information will be treated as strictly confidential and will be of great value to health professionals; there is a good chance that it may eventually benefit yourself and others with arthritis by leading to improved care and treatment.

Researchers are also experimenting with the possibility of using stem cell transplants to repair cartilage damaged by osteoarthritis.

Glossary

Acute Term describing a symptom or condition that comes on suddenly.

Analgesic A drug that relieves pain.

Antibody A protein in the blood that destroys substances or organisms that may be harmful to the body.

Anti-inflammatories Drugs, such as corticosteroids and NSAIDs, that reduce inflammation.

Antioxidants Chemicals that can neutralize free radicals.

Autoimmune Term describing a condition in which the body attacks its own tissues.

Chronic Term describing a symptom (e.g. pain) or condition (e.g. arthritis) that lasts for a long time and is slow to change.

Collagen Strong protein that forms part of cartilage and bone.

Corticosteroids Drugs that reduce inflammation by suppressing allergic responses and the immune system.

Cytokine Chemical that stimulates the immune system to combat infection.

Endorphins (encephalins) Chemicals produced by the brain and central nervous system to relieve the pain.

Enthesitis Inflammation at the point where a tendon is attached to bone.

Enzymes Proteins that increase the rate of chemical reactions in the cells of the body.

Erythrocyte Red blood cell.

Essential fatty acid Polyunsaturated fatty acids, such as omega-3, that the body needs but cannot make.

Free radicals Naturally occurring molecules that can harm the body's tissues and damage DNA, causing various health problems.

Holistic Term describing treatment of the whole person rather than just the symptoms.

Hormone Chemical with a specific function that is released directly into the bloodstream by a gland (e.g. adrenal gland) or a tissue (e.g. kidney, brain, or intestine).

Leukocyte White blood cell.

Magnetic resonance imaging A diagnostic technique that uses high-frequency radio waves to scan the internal structures of the body, especially the nervous system.

Marker Chemical or gene that indicates, but does not necessarily confirm, the presence of a condition or disorder.

Metabolism Term describing all the chemical reactions in the body, especially those that form new substances, release energy, or detoxify foreign chemicals.

Mind–body therapies Techniques and approaches that harness thoughts, feelings, imagination, and actions in order to influence a person's biochemical and structural processes.

NSAIDs Nonsteroidal anti-inflammatory drugs, which relieve painful inflammation and stiffness in muscles, joints, and bones.

Prostaglandins Synthetic or naturally occurring chemicals that can contract muscles, inflame damaged tissue, lower blood pressure, or produce mucus in the lining of the stomach.

Range of motion The normal amount that a joint can be moved in certain directions.

Supplements Nutrients, such as vitamins, minerals, and trace elements, that can be taken to supplement the diet.

Synovium The cartilage lining of a joint, which produces synovial fluid.

Tendinitis Inflammation of a tendon.

Tenosynovitis Inflammation or swelling of the sheath of tissues surrounding a tendon, enclosed within the synovial membrane.

Topical Applied to the skin.

Trace element A mineral (e.g. zinc, copper, and selenium) that the body needs in tiny amounts and can only get from digesting food.

Ultrasound A diagnostic technique that uses high-frequency sound waves to scan internal structures of the body and to treat injuries of the soft tissues.

Unsaturated fat (including polyunsaturated fat) Fat that contains fatty acids but no cholesterol.

Useful addresses

Arthritis Foundation
1330 West Peachtree Street,
Suite 100
Atlanta, GA 30309
Tel: (800) 568-4045
Tel: (404) 872-7100
Fax: (404) 872-9559
Email: help@arthritis.org
Website: www.arthritis.org
The Arthritis Foundation has 46 local
offices around the US. Enter your zip
code on the AF web site to locate the
office nearest you. Each local office
has a toll-free information line, email
and fax addresses, and information on
local programs, services, and events.
There is also a physician referral on
the website for each region.

**American Association of
Orthopaedic Medicine**
600 Pembrook Drive
Woodland Park, CO 80863
Tel: (800) 992-2063
Fax: (719) 687-5184
Email: aaom@aaomed.org
Website: www.aaom.org

**American Academy of Orthopedic
Surgeons**
6300 North River Road
Rosemont, IL 60018
Tel: (800) 346-AAOS
Tel: (847) 823-7186
Website: www.orthoinfo.aaos.org

**American Academy of Physical
Medicine and Rehabilitation**
330 North Wabash Avenue,
Suite 2500
Chicago, IL 60611
Tel: (312) 464-9700
Fax: (312) 464-0227
Email: info@aapmr.org
Website: www.aapmr.org

American College of Rheumatology
1800 Century Place
Atlanta, GA 30345
Tel: (404) 633-3777
Fax: (404) 633-1870
Email: acr@rheumatology.org
Website: www.rheumatology.org

**American Occupational Therapy
Association**
4720 Montgomery Lane
PO Box 31220
Bethesda, MD 20824
Tel: (301) 652-2682
Tel: (800) 377-8555 (TDD)
Fax: (301) 652-7711
Website: www.aota.org

**American Physical Therapy
Association**
1111 North Fairfax Street
Alexandria, VA 22314
Tel: (800) 999-APTA
Tel: (703) 684-APTA
Tel: (703) 683-6748 (TDD)
Fax: (703) 684-73434
Website: www.apta.org

**National Institute of Arthritis and
Musculoskeletal and Skin Diseases**
National Institutes of Health
Building 31, Room 4C02
31 Center Drive, MSC 2350
Bethesda, MD 20892
Tel: (301) 496-8190
Website: www.niams.nig.gov

**American Autoimmune Related
Diseases Association**
22100 Gratiot Avenue
East Detroit, MI 48021
Tel: (586) 776-3900
Website: www.aarda.org

**Centers for Disease Control
and Prevention (CDC)**
1600 Clifton Road
Atlanta, GA 30333
Tel: (800) 311-3435
Tel: (888) 232-3228
Website: www.cdc.gov

National Mental Health Association
2001 N. Beauregard Street
Alexandria, VA 22311
Tel: (800) 969-6642
Website: www.nmha.org

Aging
**American Association of Retired
People (AARP)**
601 E Street, NW
Washington, DC 20049
Tel: (800) 424-3410
Tel: (877) 434-7598 (TTY)
Email: member@aarp.org
Website: www.aarp.org

American Geriatrics Society
350 Fifth Avenue,
Suite 801
New York, NY 10118
Tel: (212) 308-1414
Email: info@americangeriatrics.org
Website: www.americangeriatrics.org

National Council on Aging
409 Third Street SW
Washington, DC 20024
Tel: (800) 424-9046
Tel: (202) 479-1200
Email: info@ncoa.org
Website: www.ncoa.org

Exercise and fitness

American Council on Exercise
4851 Paramount Drive
San Diego, CA 92123
Tel: (800) 825-3636
Tel: (858) 279-8227
Email: resource@acefitness.org
Website: www.acefitness.org

**American Council for Fitness
and Nutrition**
PO Box 33396
Washington, DC 20033
Tel: (800) 953-1700
Email: info@acfnorg
Website: www.acfm.org

Nutrition

American Dietetic Association
120 South Riverside Plaza,
Suite 2000
Chicago, IL 60606
Tel: (800) 877-1600
Website: www.eatright.org

Food and Drug Administration
5600 Fishers Lane
Rockville, MD 20857
Tel: (888) INFO-FDA
Website: www.fda.gov

Safety and health

**National Highway Traffic Safety
Association**
400 Seventh Street, SW
Washington, DC 20590
Tel: (888) 327-4236
Tel: (202) 366-0123
Website: www.nhtsa.dot.gov

National Safety Council
1121 Spring Lake Drive
Itasca, IL 60143
Tel: (630) 285-1121
Email: info@nsc.org
Website: www.nsc.org

**Occupational Safety and Health
Administration**
200 Constitutional Avenue
Washington, DC 20210
Tel: (800) 321-OSHA
Website: www.osha.org

Specific conditions

Office of Rare Diseases
National Institutes of Health
6100 Executive Boulevard
Room 3B01, MSC 7518
Bethesda, MD 20892
Tel: (301) 402-4336
Email: ord@od.nig.gov
Website: www.rarediseases.info.nih.gov

SpineUniverse.com
1737 S. Naperville Road,
Suite 203
Wheaton, IL, 60187
Website: www.spineuniverse.com

Spine-health.com
123 West Madison Street,
Suite 1450
Chicago, IL 60602
Email: admin@spine-health.com
Website: www.spine-health.com

National Fibromyalgia Association
2200 N. Glassell Street,
Suite A
Orange, CA 92865
Tel: (714) 921-0150
Fax: (714) 921-6920
Website: www.fmaware.org

**National Fibromyalgia Research
Association**
PO Box 500
Salem, OR 97308
Website: www.nfra.net

Lupus Foundation of America
1300 Piccard Drive, Suite 200
Rockville, MD 20850
Tel: (800) 558-0121
Tel: (800) 558-0231 (Spanish)
Email: lupusinfo@aol.com
Website: www.lupus.org

**American Academy of
Ophthalmology**
PO Box 7424
San Francisco, CA 94120
Tel: (415) 561-8500
Website: www.aao.org

**Foundation for Osteoporosis
Research**
300 Twenty-seventh Street,
Suite 103
Oakland, CA 94612
Tel: (888) 266-3015
Tel: (510) 832-2663
Email:info@fore.org
Website: www.fore.org

National Osteoporosis Foundation
1232 Twenty-second Street, NW
Washington, DC 20037
Tel: (202) 223-2226
Website: www.nof.org

**Osteoporosis and Related Bone
Diseases National Resource Center**
2 AMS Circle
Bethesda, MD 20892
Tel: (800) 624-BONE
Tel: (202) 223-0344
Email: NIAMSBONEINFO@mail.nih.gov
Website: www.osteo.org

Sjögren's Syndrome Foundation
8120 Woodmont Avenue, Suite 530
Bethesda, MD 20814
Tel: (800) 475-6473
Tel: (301) 718-0300
Fax: (301) 718-0322
Website: www.sjogrens.org

**Spondylitis Association
of America**
14827 Ventura Boulevard #22
Sherman Oaks, CA 91403
Tel: (800) 777-8189
Tel: (818) 981-1616
Email: info@spondylitis.org
Website: www.spondylitis.org

Children

**American Juvenile Arthritis
Foundation**
1330 West Peachtree Street,
Suite 100
Atlanta, GA 30309
Tel: (800) 568-4045
Tel: (404) 872-7100
Fax: (404) 872-9559
Email: help@arthritis.org
Website: www.arthritis.org

American Academy of Pediatrics
141 Northwest Point Boulevard
Elk Grove Village, IL 60007
Tel: (847) 434-4000
Email: kidsdocs@aap.org
Website: www.aap.org

**Federation for Children with
Special Needs**
1135 Tremont Street,
Suite 420
Boston, MA 02120
Tel: (800) 331-0688
Tel: (617) 236-7210
Fax: (617)572-2094
Email: fcsninfo@fcsn.org
Website: www.fcsn.org

KidsHealth.org
Website: www.kidshealth.org

Neymours
12735 West Gran Bay Parkway
Jacksonville, FL 32258
Tel: (866) 390-3610
Website: www.nemours.org

Complementary therapies

American Chiropractic Association
1701 Clarendon Boulevard
Arlington, VA 22209
Tel: (800) 986-4636
Email: memberinfo@amerchiro.org
Website: www.amerchiro.org

**American Massage Therapy
Associationl**
500 Davis Street, Suite 900
Evanston, IL 60201
Tel: (847) 864-0123
Tel: (877) 905-2700
Email: info@amtamassage.org
Website: www.amtamassage.org

**American Academy of Medical
Acupuncture**
4929 Wilshire Boulevard,
Suite 428
Los Angeles, CA 90010
Tel: (323) 937-5514
Website: www.medicalacupuncture.org

American Academy of Osteopathy
3500 DePauw Bolevard, Suite 1080
Indianapolis, IN 46268
Tel: (317) 879-1881
Website: www.academyofosteopathy.org

**American Herbal Products
Association**
8484 Georgia Avenue, Suite 370
Silver Spring, MD 20910
(301) 588-1171
Email: ahpa@ahpa.org
Website: www.ahpa.org

**American Society for the
Alexander Technique**
PO Box 60008
Florence, MA 01062
Tel: (800) 473-0620
Tel: (413) 584-2359
Email: info@amsat.ws
Website: www.alexandertech.com

The American Tai Chi Association
2465 J-17 Centreville Road,
Suite 150
Herndon, VA 20171
Email: contact@americantaichi.net
Website: www.americantaichi.net

**National Certification Commission
for Acupuncture and Oriental
Medicine**
11 Canal Center Plaza,
Suite 300
Tel: (703) 548-9004
Email: info@nccaom.org
Website: www.nccaom.org

Register of Chinese Herbal Medicine
PO Box 162340
Sacramento, CA 95816
Tel: (916) 443-4770
Email: info@aaom.org
Website: www.aaom.org

Pain

American Chronic Pain Association
PO Box 850
Rocklin, CA 95677
Tel: (800) 533-3231
Email: ACPA@pacbell.net
Website: www.theacpa.org

American Pain Foundation
201 N. Charles Street,
Suite 710
Baltimore, MD 21201
Tel: (888) 615-PAIN
Website: www.painfoundation.org

**National Chronic Pain Outreach
Association**
PO Box 274
Millboro, VA 24460
Tel: (540) 862-9437
Website: www.chronicpain.org

Index

About the authors

David L Scott is Professor of Clinical Rheumatology at King's College Hospital, London. Howard Bird is Professor of Pharmacological Rheumatology at the University of Leeds. Andrew Hamer is Consultant Orthopedic Surgeon at the Northern General Hospital, Sheffield.

Alison Hammond is Senior Lecturer in Rheumatology at the University of Brighton and Rheumatology Research Therapist in Derby. Mike Hurley is Reader in Physiotherapy at King's College London. Dorothy Pattison is Lecturer in Dietetics at the University of Plymouth. Janet Harkess

is Clinical Specialist Occupational Therapist based in Fife. Paula Jeffreson is a Specialist Occupational Therapist in Rheumatology based in Shropshire. Caroline Green is a freelance health writer with a special interest in arthritis and complementary therapies.

Acknowledgments

DK Publishing would like to thank the following people: Trina Alcorn and Susan Bernstein of the Arthritis Foundation for their assistance in obtaining arthritis prevalence statistics. Christine Edwards, Kate Llewelyn, Jo Cumming, and the

Helpline team at Arthritis Care for their expert review and advice. Ann Baggaley for contributing to several chapters, and for proofreading the British edition. Jane Perlmutter for proofreading the US edition. The Food Standards Agency for

information on salt and fat labeling, and the alcoholic content of some drinks. Ruth Jenkinson for new photography. Pat Perse-White and Ann Greenhouse for modeling. Roisin Donaghy for hair and makeup. Hilary Bird for the index.

Picture credits

Alamy: John Angerson 65, Buzz Pictures 69, ImageState 142, Black Star 198.
Corbis: Norbert Schaefe 2, Randy Faris 7, Larry Williams 8, Ariel Skelley 16, JLP/Sylvia Torres/Zefa 32, Tom & Dee Ann McCarthy 35, LWA-Dann Tardif 43, Tim Pannell 45, LWA-Stephen Welstead 46, Tom Stewart 47, JLP/Jose L. Pelaez 50, Richard Cummins 57, Michael Keller 59, PhotoCuisine 61, Chuck Savage 64, Chuck Savage 67, Paul Barton 70, Ariel Skelley 71, Helen King 72, Tom & Dee Ann McCarthy 73tr, Jose Luis Pelaez, Inc. 77, A. Inden/Zefa 98, Helen King 101, Rolf Bruderer 104, Kelly-Mooney Photography 107, Tom Stewart 132, Walter Hodges 143, David Stoeklein 146, Tom & Dee Ann McCarthy 149, Strauss/Curtis 151, Thomas Schweizer 152, Norbert Schaefer 153, Gabe Palmer 154, Jim Craigmyle 156, Bob Krist 157, Simon Taplin 158, Chuck Savage 159,

John Henley 173, Randy Faris 180, Tract Kahn 182, Randy Faris 185, Randy Faris 186, Tom Stewart 187, Simon Marcus 189, Tim Pannell 192, Rolf Bruderer 195tl, Jim Cummins 197, Gabe Palmer 201, Mark A. Johnson 202, George Shelley 204, Paul Barton 206, Randy Faris 207, Tom & Dee Ann McCarthy 208. **Getty Images:** Andre Cezar 52. **Andrew Hamer** 95.
Mediscan 130. **Photolibrary.com:** Mauritius Die Bildagentur Gmbh 11, Bsip 26, Aflo Foto Agency 30, Workbook, Inc. 36, Bsip 39tr, Phototake Inc. 40, Phototake Inc 42, Simon Smith Photography Ltd 63, Phototake Inc 73br, Phototake Inc 74, Mauritius Die Bildagentur Gmbh 76, Bsip 78, Bsip 80, Bsip 86, Bsip 88, Mode Images ltd 103, Phototake Inc 110, Foodpix 118, Phototake Inc 120, Pacific Stock 128, Bsip 134, Photononstop 175,

It Stock 191, Workbook, Inc. 195br, Bsip196. **Science Photo Library:** Science Photo Library 6, Zephyr 14, Princess Margaret Rose Orthopaedic Hospital 17, Science Photo Library 19, CNRI 21, Eye Of Science 25, Dr. P. Marazzi 27, CNRI 34, Simon Fraser, Royal Victoria Infirmary 39br, Bsip, LBL 41, Dr. P. Marazzi 83, Prof. P. Motta / Dept. of Anatomy / University "La Sapienza", Rome 193tr, Hybrid Medical Animation 193br, AJ Photo 209, AJ Photo 210, Professor Miodrag Stojkovic 211, Philippe Plailly / Eurelios 212.
Superstock: SuperStock, Inc. 10, Powerstock 48, Florian Franke 172, Age Fotostock 188, Age Fotostock 190 **Mike Wyndham** 31, 38

All other images © **Dorling Kindersley:** For further information see **www. dkimages.com**